Pegan Diet Cookbook for Beginners

1000-Days of Mouthwatering,Delicious Recipes, Meal Plans, and Practical Tips for Beginners to Achieve Optimal Health and Sustainable Weight Loss

By Tori Aarya

TABLE OF CONTENTS

INTRODUCTION

Welcome to the "Pegan Diet Cookbook for Beginners: 1000-Days of Mouthwatering, Delicious Recipes, Meal Plans, and Practical Tips for Beginners to Achieve Optimal Health and Sustainable Weight Loss." In this cookbook, we will embark on an exciting culinary journey that combines the best of two popular eating approaches: the Paleo and vegan diets. By adopting a Pegan diet, you'll have the opportunity to enhance your health, enjoy delicious meals, and achieve sustainable weight loss.

In recent years, the Paleo and vegan diets have gained significant attention for their respective health benefits. The Paleo diet, inspired by the eating habits of our ancestors, focuses on whole, unprocessed foods and eliminates grains, dairy, and legumes. On the other hand, the vegan diet excludes all animal products, promoting a plant-based lifestyle centred around fruits, vegetables, grains, legumes, and nuts.

The Pegan diet aims to balance these two approaches, combining the best elements to create a flexible and nutritious eating plan. By following the Pegan diet, you can harness the power of nutrient-dense foods while enjoying a wide variety of flavours and culinary delights.

In this cookbook, we have compiled an extensive collection of mouthwatering recipes specifically designed for beginners. Whether you're new to the Pegan diet or simply looking for fresh and exciting recipes, this cookbook will be your ultimate guide. From hearty breakfasts and nourishing salads to satisfying main courses and delectable desserts, we have included a diverse range of recipes to suit every palate and occasion.

Additionally, we understand that adopting a new eating plan can be challenging, so we have provided practical tips and guidance throughout the cookbook. You'll find helpful advice on meal planning, grocery shopping, food substitutions, and maintaining a balanced Pegan lifestyle. We aim to support you on your journey towards optimal health and sustainable weight loss by providing you with the tools and knowledge needed to succeed.

Remember, the Pegan diet is not about strict rules or deprivation; it's about nourishing your body with wholesome, nutrient-rich foods while enjoying the pleasures of eating. So, get ready to embark on a culinary adventure that will improve your health and tantalize your taste buds.

We hope this "Pegan Diet Cookbook for Beginners" becomes your trusted companion, inspiring you to explore the world of Pegan cooking and empowering you to achieve optimal health and sustainable weight loss. Let's begin this exciting journey together!

Happy cooking and bon appétit!

Note: Before making any significant dietary changes, it is always advisable to consult with a healthcare professional or registered dietitian to ensure the Pegan diet is suitable for your individual needs and health goals.

2-WEEK MEAL PLAN

WEEK 1:

Day 1: Breakfast: Scrambled tofu with vegetables (spinach, bell peppers, onions) cooked in olive oil. Lunch: Mixed green salad with grilled chicken, avocado, cherry tomatoes, and a lemon-tahini dressing. Dinner: Baked salmon with roasted Brussels sprouts and sweet potatoes. Snack: Almonds and blueberries.

Day 2: Breakfast: Chia seed pudding made with almond milk, topped with sliced almonds and berries. Lunch: Quinoa and black bean salad with diced vegetables (cucumber, tomatoes, red onion) and a lime-cilantro dressing. Dinner: Zucchini noodles (zoodles) with marinara sauce, sautéed mushrooms, and lentil meatballs. Snack: Carrot sticks with hummus.

Day 3: Breakfast: Mixed berry smoothie with almond milk, spinach, chia seeds, and a scoop of plant-based protein powder. Lunch: Roasted vegetable and chickpea wrap with whole-grain tortilla, avocado, and a drizzle of tahini sauce. Dinner: Grilled chicken breast with steamed broccoli and cauliflower rice. Snack: Apple slices with almond butter.

Day 4: Breakfast: Avocado and tomato on whole-grain toast. Lunch: Lentil soup with a side of mixed green salad. Dinner: Baked cod with asparagus and quinoa. Snack: Celery sticks with almond butter.

Day 5: Breakfast: Vegetable omelette made with bell peppers, onions, mushrooms, and spinach. Lunch: Greek salad with mixed greens, cucumbers, cherry tomatoes, olives, and tofu feta cheese. Dinner: Stir-fried tofu with bok choy, snap peas, and brown rice. Snack: Mixed nuts and seeds.

Day 6: Breakfast: Banana and almond butter smoothie with a handful of spinach. Lunch: Roasted sweet potato and black bean bowl with avocado, salsa, and cilantro. Dinner: Grilled shrimp skewers with grilled vegetables (zucchini, bell peppers, onions) and quinoa. Snack: Sliced cucumbers with guacamole.

Day 7: Breakfast: Coconut milk yoghurt topped with sliced almonds, coconut flakes, and fresh berries. Lunch: Quinoa tabbouleh salad with diced cucumbers, cherry tomatoes, parsley, and lemon dressing. Dinner: Baked chicken thighs with roasted root vegetables (carrots, parsnips, turnips). Snack: Roasted chickpeas.

WEEK 2:

Repeat the meal plan from Week 1, or mix and match your favourite recipes from the previous week to create a variety of meals.

Remember to stay hydrated throughout the day by drinking water and herbal tea. You can adjust the recipes and ingredients based on your preferences and dietary restrictions. Enjoy your Pegan diet journey!

ROASTED CAULIFLOWER STEAKS WITH CHIMICHURRI SAUCE

Preparation Time: 15 minutes Cooking Time: 25 minutes Serving: 4 servings

Ingredients:

- One large head of cauliflower
- Three tablespoons olive oil
- Salt and black pepper, to taste
- For the Chimichurri Sauce:
    - 1 cup fresh parsley leaves, finely chopped
    - 1/4 cup fresh cilantro leaves, finely chopped
    - Three cloves garlic, minced
    - 1/4 cup red wine vinegar
    - 1/2 cup extra virgin olive oil
    - One teaspoon of dried oregano
    - 1/2 teaspoon red pepper flakes
    - Salt and black pepper, to taste

Directions:

1. Preheat your oven to 425°F (220°C). Line a baking sheet with parchment paper or lightly grease it.

2. Remove the leaves from the cauliflower head and trim the stem so that the cauliflower sits flat on a cutting board. Slice the

cauliflower into 1-inch thick steaks, starting from the centre. You should be able to get 3 to 4 steaks from a large head of cauliflower. Save any florets that break off for another use.

3. Place the cauliflower steaks on the prepared baking sheet. Drizzle with olive oil and season with salt and black pepper to taste. Use your hands or a brush to ensure the steaks are evenly coated with oil.

4. Roast the cauliflower steaks in the preheated oven for about 20-25 minutes or until they are tender and golden brown around the edges.

5. While the cauliflower is roasting, prepare the chimichurri sauce. In a bowl, combine the parsley, cilantro, minced garlic, red wine vinegar, extra virgin olive oil, dried oregano, and red pepper flakes. Season with salt and black pepper to taste. Stir well to combine all the ingredients.

6. Once the cauliflower steaks are done, remove them from the oven and let them cool slightly. Serve the steaks with a generous drizzle of chimichurri sauce on top.

Nutrition Facts (per serving):

- Calories: 187
- Fat: 17g
- Saturated Fat: 2g
- Sodium: 160mg
- Carbohydrates: 7g
- Fibre: 3g
- Sugar: 3g
- Protein: 2g

Note: The nutrition facts may vary depending on the specific ingredients and quantities used.

QUINOA AND LENTIL STUFFED PEPPERS

Preparation Time: 15 minutes Cooking Time: 45 minutes Serving: 4 servings

Ingredients:

- Four large bell peppers (any colour)
- 1 cup cooked quinoa
- 1 cup cooked lentils
- One small onion, finely chopped
- Two cloves garlic, minced
- One carrot, grated
- One celery stalk, finely chopped
- 1 cup diced tomatoes
- One teaspoon of dried oregano
- One teaspoon of dried basil
- 1/2 teaspoon cumin
- Salt and pepper to taste
- 1/2 cup shredded mozzarella cheese (optional)
- Fresh parsley, chopped (for garnish)

Directions:

1. Preheat the oven to 375°F (190°C).

2. Cut off the tops of the bell peppers and remove the seeds and membranes. Rinse them well.

3. In a large mixing bowl, combine the cooked quinoa, lentils, onion, garlic, carrot, celery, diced tomatoes, dried oregano, dried basil, cumin, salt, and pepper. Mix well to combine.

4. Stuff each bell pepper with the quinoa and lentil mixture, packing it tightly. Place the stuffed peppers upright in a baking dish.

5. If desired, sprinkle shredded mozzarella cheese over each stuffed pepper.

6. Cover the baking dish with foil and bake in the oven for 30 minutes.

7. Remove the foil and bake for an additional 10-15 minutes, or until the peppers are tender and the cheese is melted and bubbly.

8. Remove from the oven and let the stuffed peppers cool for a few minutes. Garnish with fresh chopped parsley before serving.

Nutrition Facts (per serving):

- Calories: 220
- Total Fat: 3g
- Saturated Fat: 1g
- Cholesterol: 5mg
- Sodium: 220mg
- Total Carbohydrate: 38g
- Dietary Fiber: 11g
- Sugars: 7g
- Protein: 12g

Note: Nutrition facts may vary depending on the specific ingredients and brands used.

SPAGHETTI SQUASH PAD THAI

Preparation Time: 15 minutes Cooking Time: 30 minutes Serving: 4 servings

Ingredients:

- One medium-sized spaghetti squash
- Two tablespoons of vegetable oil
- One small onion, finely chopped
- 2 cloves garlic, minced
- 1 red bell pepper, thinly sliced
- One carrot, julienned
- 1 cup bean sprouts
- 2 green onions, chopped
- 1/4 cup roasted peanuts, chopped (optional)
- Fresh cilantro leaves for garnish

For the Pad Thai Sauce:

- Three tablespoons soy sauce
- Two tablespoons of lime juice
- Two tablespoons tamarind paste

- Two tablespoons brown sugar
- One tablespoon fish sauce (optional for non-vegetarian version)
- One teaspoon sriracha sauce (adjust to taste)

Directions:

1. Preheat your oven to 400°F (200°C). Cut the spaghetti squash in half lengthwise and scoop out the seeds. Place the squash halves on a baking sheet, cut side up. Bake in the preheated oven for 25-30 minutes or until the squash is tender. Once cooked, remove it from the oven and let it cool for a few minutes.

2. While the squash is cooking, prepare the Pad Thai sauce. In a small bowl, whisk together the soy sauce, lime juice, tamarind paste, brown sugar, fish sauce (if using), and sriracha sauce. Set aside.

3. Heat the vegetable oil in a large skillet or wok over medium-high heat. Add the onion and garlic, and sauté for 2-3 minutes until fragrant and translucent.

4. Add the red bell pepper, carrot, and bean sprouts to the skillet. Stir-fry for another 3-4 minutes until the vegetables are tender-crisp.

5. Using a fork, scrape the flesh of the cooked spaghetti squash into the skillet with the vegetables. Toss everything together until well combined.

6. Pour the Pad Thai sauce over the mixture in the skillet. Stir-fry for an additional 2-3 minutes to allow the flavours to meld together.

7. Remove the skillet from the heat and garnish with chopped green onions and roasted peanuts (if using). Serve the Spaghetti Squash Pad Thai hot, garnished with fresh cilantro leaves.

Nutrition Facts (per serving):

- Calories: 220
- Fat: 10g
- Saturated Fat: 1.5g
- Sodium: 700mg
- Carbohydrates: 30g
- Fibre: 5g
- Sugar: 15g
- Protein: 6g

Note: The nutrition facts provided are approximate and may vary based on the specific ingredients used.

SWEET POTATO AND BLACK BEAN ENCHILADAS

Preparation Time: 20 minutes Cooking Time: 40 minutes Serving: 4 servings

Ingredients:

- Two large sweet potatoes, peeled and diced
- One can (15 ounces) of black beans, rinsed and drained
- One small onion, finely chopped
- Two cloves garlic, minced
- One tablespoon of olive oil

- One teaspoon of ground cumin
- One teaspoon of chilli powder
- 1/2 teaspoon smoked paprika
- Salt and pepper to taste
- One can (15 ounces) of enchilada sauce
- Eight small flour tortillas
- 1 cup shredded cheese (cheddar or Mexican blend)
- Chopped fresh cilantro for garnish (optional)
- Sour cream for serving (optional)

Directions:

1. Preheat your oven to 375°F (190°C).

2. heat the olive oil over medium heat in a large skillet. Add the onion and garlic, and sauté until the onion is translucent and fragrant, about 2-3 minutes.

3. Add the diced sweet potatoes to the skillet and cook for about 10 minutes, stirring occasionally, until tender.

4. Add the black beans, cumin, chilli powder, smoked paprika, salt, and pepper to the skillet. Stir well to combine all the ingredients and cook for an additional 2-3 minutes.

5. Pour about 1/3 cup of enchilada sauce into the bottom of a baking dish.

6. Place a tortilla on a clean surface and spoon about 1/4 cup of the sweet potato and black bean mixture onto the centre of the tortilla. Roll it up tightly and place it seam-side down in the baking dish. Repeat this process with the remaining tortillas and filling.

7. Pour the remaining enchilada sauce over the rolled tortillas, ensuring they are all coated. Sprinkle the shredded cheese evenly over the top.

8. Cover the baking dish with foil and bake in the preheated oven for 25 minutes. Then, remove the foil and bake for 10-15 minutes until the cheese is bubbly and lightly browned.

9. Once cooked, remove the enchiladas from the oven and let them cool for a few minutes. Garnish with chopped cilantro, if desired.

10. Serve the Sweet Potato and Black Bean Enchiladas warm, with a dollop of sour cream on top if you like. Enjoy!

Nutrition Facts (per serving):

- Calories: 410
- Fat: 13g
- Carbohydrates: 61g
- Fibre: 11g
- Protein: 15g
- Sugar: 8g
- Sodium: 860mg

Note: Nutrition facts may vary depending on the specific ingredients and brands used.

MUSHROOM AND SPINACH STUFFED PORTOBELLO MUSHROOMS

Preparation Time: 15 minutes

Cooking Time: 25 minutes

Serving: 4 servings

Ingredients:

- Four large Portobello mushrooms
- 2 tablespoons olive oil
- Two cloves garlic, minced
- One small onion, finely chopped
- 2 cups baby spinach, chopped
- 1 cup mushrooms, finely chopped
- 1/2 cup breadcrumbs
- 1/2 cup grated Parmesan cheese
- 1/2 teaspoon dried thyme
- Salt and pepper to taste

Directions:

1. Preheat the oven to 375°F (190°C). Clean the Portobello mushrooms and remove the stems. Place them on a baking sheet, gill side up.

2. In a skillet, heat the olive oil over medium heat. Add the garlic and onion, and sauté until softened and fragrant, about 3 minutes.

3. Add the baby spinach and chopped mushrooms to the skillet. Cook until the spinach wilts and the mushrooms release their moisture, about 5 minutes. Remove from heat.

4. In a bowl, combine the cooked spinach and mushrooms with breadcrumbs, Parmesan cheese, dried thyme, salt, and pepper. Stir well to combine.

5. Divide the stuffing mixture evenly among the Portobello mushrooms, filling the caps generously.

6. Bake the stuffed mushrooms in the preheated oven for about 20 minutes or until the mushrooms are tender and the stuffing is golden brown.

7. Once cooked, remove from the oven and let them cool slightly before serving.

Nutrition Facts (per serving):

- Calories: 170
- Fat: 10g
- Carbohydrates: 13g
- Protein: 8g
- Fibre: 3g

Enjoy your delicious Mushroom and Spinach Stuffed Portobello Mushrooms!

COCONUT CURRY LENTIL SOUP

Preparation Time: 15 minutes Cooking Time: 30 minutes Serving: 4

Ingredients:

- One tablespoon of coconut oil
- One medium onion, chopped
- Three cloves garlic, minced
- One tablespoon of fresh ginger, grated
- Two tablespoons of curry powder
- One teaspoon of ground cumin
- 1 cup red lentils
- 4 cups vegetable broth
- One can (14 ounces) of coconut milk
- 1 cup diced tomatoes (canned or fresh)
- 1 cup chopped spinach or kale
- Juice of 1 lime
- Salt and pepper to taste
- Fresh cilantro for garnish (optional)

Directions:

1. Heat the coconut oil in a large pot over medium heat. Add the chopped onion and sauté until translucent, about 5 minutes.

2. Add the minced garlic and grated ginger to the pot and sauté for another minute until fragrant.

3. Stir in the curry powder and ground cumin, coating the onions, garlic, and ginger with the spices.

4. Add the red lentils to the pot and stir to combine with the spice mixture.

5. Pour in the vegetable broth and bring the mixture to a boil. Reduce the heat to low, cover the pot, and simmer for 20 minutes or until the lentils are tender.

6. Stir in the coconut milk, diced tomatoes, and chopped spinach or kale. Cook for an additional 5 minutes until the vegetables are wilted and heated through.

7. Remove the pot from heat and stir in the lime juice. Season with salt and pepper to taste.

8. Ladle the Coconut Curry Lentil Soup into serving bowls and garnish with fresh cilantro, if desired.

9. Serve hot, and enjoy!

Nutrition Facts (per serving):

- Calories: 320
- Fat: 17g
- Saturated Fat: 14g
- Carbohydrates: 35g
- Fibre: 11g
- Sugar: 5g
- Protein: 11g
- Sodium: 800mg

Note: Nutrition facts are approximate and may vary depending on the ingredients used.

ALMOND CRUSTED BAKED CHICKEN

Preparation Time: 15 minutes Cooking Time: 25 minutes Serving: 4 servings

Ingredients:

- Four boneless, skinless chicken breasts
- 1 cup almonds, finely ground
- 1/2 cup breadcrumbs
- 1/4 cup grated Parmesan cheese
- One teaspoon of dried thyme
- One teaspoon paprika
- 1/2 teaspoon salt
- 1/4 teaspoon black pepper
- Two large eggs, beaten
- Cooking spray or olive oil

Directions:

1. Preheat your oven to 400°F (200°C). Line a baking sheet with parchment paper or lightly grease it with cooking spray or olive oil.

2. In a shallow dish or plate, combine the ground almonds, breadcrumbs, Parmesan cheese, dried thyme, paprika, salt, and black pepper. Mix well.

3. Dip each chicken breast into the beaten eggs, allowing any excess to drip off. Then, coat the chicken breasts in the almond mixture, pressing it onto both sides to adhere.

4. Place the coated chicken breasts on the prepared baking sheet. If desired, lightly spray the top of the chicken with cooking spray or drizzle with a little olive oil for extra crispiness.

5. Bake in the preheated oven for 20-25 minutes or until the chicken is cooked and the crust is golden brown. The internal temperature of the chicken should reach 165°F (74°C).

6. Once cooked, remove the chicken from the oven and let it rest for a few minutes before serving.

Nutrition Facts (per serving):

- Calories: 320
- Fat: 15g
- Saturated Fat: 3g
- Cholesterol: 160mg
- Sodium: 570mg
- Carbohydrates: 9g
- Fibre: 3g
- Sugar: 1g
- Protein: 38g

Note: Nutrition facts are approximate and may vary depending on the ingredients used.

MEDITERRANEAN CHICKPEA SALAD

Preparation Time: 15 minutes Cooking Time: 0 minutes Serving: 4 servings

Ingredients:

- Two cans (15 ounces each) of chickpeas, drained and rinsed
- 1 English cucumber, diced
- One red bell pepper, diced
- 1/2 red onion, thinly sliced
- 1 cup cherry tomatoes, halved
- 1/2 cup Kalamata olives, pitted and halved
- 1/2 cup crumbled feta cheese
- 1/4 cup fresh parsley, chopped
- 1/4 cup fresh mint leaves, chopped

For the dressing:

- 1/4 cup extra-virgin olive oil
- Two tablespoons of lemon juice
- Two cloves garlic, minced
- One teaspoon of dried oregano
- Salt and pepper to taste

Directions:

1. In a large bowl, combine the chickpeas, cucumber, bell pepper, red onion, cherry tomatoes, Kalamata olives, feta cheese, parsley, and mint leaves.

2. In a separate small bowl, whisk together the olive oil, lemon juice, minced garlic, dried oregano, salt, and pepper until well combined.

3. Pour the dressing over the salad ingredients and toss gently to coat everything evenly.

4. Let the salad sit for about 10 minutes to allow the flavours to meld together.

5. Serve the Mediterranean Chickpea Salad chilled or at room temperature. It can be enjoyed on its own as a light meal or as a side dish with grilled chicken, fish, or crusty bread.

Nutrition Facts (per serving):

- Calories: 320
- Fat: 18g
- Carbohydrates: 32g
- Fibre: 8g
- Protein: 10g
- Sodium: 610mg
- Sugar: 6g

Note: The nutrition facts provided are approximate and may vary based on the specific ingredients used.

ZUCCHINI NOODLES WITH AVOCADO PESTO

Preparation Time: 15 minutes Cooking Time: 0 minutes Serving: 2 servings

Ingredients:

- Two medium-sized zucchinis
- One ripe avocado
- 1/2 cup fresh basil leaves
- 1/4 cup pine nuts

- Two cloves garlic, minced
- Juice of 1 lemon
- Two tablespoons extra-virgin olive oil
- Salt and pepper to taste
- Optional toppings: cherry tomatoes, grated Parmesan cheese

Directions:

1. Wash the zucchinis and trim off the ends. Using a spiralizer or julienne peeler, create zucchini noodles and set them aside in a bowl.
2. In a food processor, combine the avocado, basil leaves, pine nuts, minced garlic, lemon juice, olive oil, salt, and pepper. Blend until smooth and creamy, adjusting the seasoning to taste.
3. Pour the avocado pesto over the zucchini noodles and toss gently until the noodles are evenly coated.
4. Optional: If desired, top the zucchini noodles with halved cherry tomatoes and a sprinkle of grated Parmesan cheese.
5. Serve the zucchini noodles immediately, either chilled or at room temperature.

Nutrition Facts (per serving):

- Calories: 230
- Fat: 19g
- Carbohydrates: 12g
- Fibre: 8g
- Protein: 5g
- Vitamin C: 30% DV
- Vitamin A: 15% DV

- Calcium: 4% DV
- Iron: 8% DV

Note: The nutrition facts are approximate and may vary depending on the ingredients used.

ROASTED BRUSSELS SPROUTS WITH BALSAMIC GLAZE

Preparation Time: 10 minutes Cooking Time: 25 minutes Serving: 4

Ingredients:

- 1 pound Brussels sprouts, trimmed and halved
- Two tablespoons of olive oil
- Salt and pepper to taste
- Two tablespoons of balsamic vinegar
- One tablespoon honey
- Two cloves garlic, minced

Directions:

1. Preheat your oven to 425°F (220°C).
2. In a large bowl, combine the Brussels sprouts, olive oil, salt, and pepper. Toss them together until the sprouts are evenly coated.
3. Spread the Brussels sprouts out in a single layer on a baking sheet. Make sure they are evenly spaced for better roasting.
4. Place the baking sheet in the preheated oven and roast the Brussels sprouts for about 20-25 minutes or until they are tender

and nicely browned, stirring once or twice during the cooking process for even browning.

5. While the Brussels sprouts are roasting, prepare the balsamic glaze. Combine the balsamic vinegar, honey, and minced garlic in a small saucepan. Heat the mixture over medium heat, stirring occasionally, until it thickens and reduces to a glaze-like consistency. This should take about 5-7 minutes. Remove from heat.

6. Once the Brussels sprouts are roasted, transfer them to a serving dish. Drizzle the balsamic glaze over the roasted sprouts, tossing gently to ensure they are coated evenly.

7. Serve the roasted Brussels sprouts with balsamic glaze immediately as a side dish or a light snack.

Nutrition Facts (per serving):

- Calories: 120
- Total Fat: 7g
- Saturated Fat: 1g
- Sodium: 50mg
- Total Carbohydrate: 13g
- Dietary Fiber: 4g
- Sugars: 6g
- Protein: 4g
- Vitamin C: 120% DV
- Iron: 10% DV

Note: The nutrition facts are approximate and may vary based on the specific ingredients used.

BAKED SALMON WITH LEMON-DILL SAUCE

Preparation Time: 10 minutes Cooking Time: 20 minutes Serving: 4 servings

Ingredients:

- Four salmon fillets (6 ounces each)
- One lemon, sliced
- Salt and pepper to taste
- One tablespoon of olive oil

For the Lemon-Dill Sauce:

- 1/2 cup mayonnaise
- One tablespoon of lemon juice
- One tablespoon of chopped fresh dill
- One clove of garlic, minced
- Salt and pepper to taste

Directions:

1. Preheat the oven to 400°F (200°C). Line a baking sheet with parchment paper.
2. Place the salmon fillets on the prepared baking sheet. Season each fillet with salt and pepper to taste. Arrange lemon slices on top of each fillet.
3. Drizzle the olive oil over the salmon fillets.
4. Bake the salmon in the preheated oven for about 15-20 minutes or until cooked through and flakes easily with a fork.

5. While the salmon is baking, prepare the lemon-dill sauce. In a small bowl, combine the mayonnaise, lemon juice, chopped dill, minced garlic, salt, and pepper. Mix well until fully combined.

6. Once the salmon is cooked, remove it from the oven and let it cool for a few minutes.

7. Serve the baked salmon with a dollop of lemon-dill sauce on top.

8. You can also serve the salmon with your choice of side dishes, such as roasted vegetables or a salad.

Nutrition Facts (per serving):

- Calories: 380
- Fat: 28g
- Saturated Fat: 4g
- Cholesterol: 95mg
- Sodium: 320mg
- Carbohydrates: 2g
- Fibre: 0g
- Sugar: 1g
- Protein: 31g

Note: Nutrition facts may vary depending on the specific ingredients and quantities used.

CAULIFLOWER FRIED RICE

Preparation Time: 15 minutes Cooking Time: 15 minutes Serving: 4

Ingredients:

- One medium-sized cauliflower head
- Two tablespoons of vegetable oil
- Two cloves garlic, minced
- One small onion, finely chopped
- One carrot, diced
- 1/2 cup frozen peas
- Two eggs, lightly beaten
- Three tablespoons soy sauce
- One tablespoon of oyster sauce (optional)
- 1/2 teaspoon sesame oil
- Salt and pepper to taste
- Green onions, chopped (for garnish)

Directions:

1. Cut the cauliflower into florets and discard the tough stem. Place the florets in a food processor and pulse until they resemble rice grains. Be careful not to over-process and turn it into a puree. Set aside.

2. Heat one tablespoon of vegetable oil in a large skillet or wok over medium-high heat. Add the minced garlic and chopped onion, and sauté for 2-3 minutes until fragrant, and the onion becomes translucent.

3. Add the diced carrot and frozen peas to the skillet. Stir-fry for another 2 minutes until the vegetables are tender-crisp.

4. Push the vegetables to one side of the skillet and add the beaten eggs to the other. Scramble the eggs until cooked through, then mix them with the vegetables.

5. add another tablespoon of vegetable oil and cauliflower rice in the same skillet. Stir-fry for about 5 minutes until the cauliflower is tender.

6. Add the soy sauce, oyster sauce (if using), sesame oil, salt, and pepper to the skillet. Stir-fry for another 2 minutes, ensuring the sauce is evenly distributed, and the cauliflower is well coated.

7. Remove from heat and garnish with chopped green onions.

8. Serve the cauliflower fried rice hot as a delicious and healthy alternative to regular fried rice.

Nutrition Facts (per serving):

- Calories: 150
- Total Fat: 8g
- Saturated Fat: 1g
- Cholesterol: 93mg
- Sodium: 680mg
- Total Carbohydrate: 14g
- Dietary Fiber: 4g
- Sugars: 6g
- Protein: 7g

Note: Nutrition facts may vary depending on the specific brands and quantities of ingredients used.

LENTIL AND VEGETABLE CURRY

Preparation Time: 15 minutes Cooking Time: 30 minutes Serving: 4

Ingredients:

- 1 cup lentils (any variety), rinsed and drained
- Two tablespoons of vegetable oil
- One large onion, chopped
- Three cloves garlic, minced
- One tablespoon of grated ginger
- One teaspoon of ground cumin
- One teaspoon of ground coriander
- 1/2 teaspoon turmeric
- 1/2 teaspoon chilli powder (adjust to taste)
- 2 cups chopped mixed vegetables (such as carrots, bell peppers, and zucchini)
- One can (400 grams) of diced tomatoes
- One can (400 ml) of coconut milk
- Salt to taste
- Fresh cilantro, chopped (for garnish)
- Cooked rice or naan bread (for serving)

Directions:

1. In a large pot, bring water to a boil and add the lentils. Cook them until tender but not mushy, about 15 minutes. Drain and set aside.

2. In a separate large pot, heat the vegetable oil over medium heat. Add the chopped onion and cook until it becomes translucent about 5 minutes.

3. Add the minced garlic and grated ginger to the pot and sauté for another 2 minutes until fragrant.

4. Stir in the ground cumin, coriander, turmeric, and chilli powder. Cook the spices for 1 minute to release their flavours.

5. Add the chopped mixed vegetables to the pot and cook for 5 minutes, stirring occasionally.

6. Pour in the diced tomatoes with their juice and the coconut milk. Stir well to combine all the ingredients.

7. Season with salt to taste and bring the curry to a simmer. Let it cook for 15-20 minutes or until the vegetables are tender.

8. Add the cooked lentils to the pot and stir to combine. Simmer for an additional 5 minutes to allow the flavours to meld together.

9. Taste and adjust the seasoning if needed.

10. Serve the Lentil and Vegetable Curry over cooked rice or with warm naan bread. Garnish with fresh chopped cilantro.

Nutrition Facts (per serving):

- Calories: 350
- Fat: 20g
- Carbohydrates: 35g
- Fibre: 12g
- Protein: 10g

Note: The nutrition facts provided are approximate and may vary based on the specific ingredients used.

VEGAN BLACK BEAN CHILI

Preparation Time: 15 minutes Cooking Time: 40 minutes Serving: 4-6 servings

Ingredients:

- Two tablespoons of olive oil
- One large onion, chopped
- Three cloves garlic, minced
- One red bell pepper, diced
- One green bell pepper, diced
- Two medium carrots, diced
- One jalapeño pepper, seeded and minced (optional, for heat)
- Two tablespoons chilli powder
- One tablespoon of ground cumin
- One teaspoon of smoked paprika
- One teaspoon of dried oregano
- One can (15 ounces) of diced tomatoes
- Two cans (15 ounces each) of black beans, rinsed and drained
- One can (15 ounces) of corn kernels, drained
- 2 cups vegetable broth

- Salt and pepper to taste
- Fresh cilantro, chopped (for garnish)
- Lime wedges (for serving)

Directions:

1. Heat the olive oil in a large pot or Dutch oven over medium heat. Add the onion, garlic, bell peppers, carrots, and jalapeño (if using). Sauté for about 5 minutes until the vegetables start to soften.

2. Stir in the chilli powder, cumin, smoked paprika, and oregano.

3. Add the diced tomatoes, black beans, corn, and vegetable broth to the pot. Stir well to combine all the ingredients. Bring the mixture to a boil, then reduce the heat to low and cover the pot.

4. Simmer the chilli for about 30 minutes, stirring occasionally. If the chilli becomes too thick, add more vegetable broth or water to reach your desired consistency.

5. Season with salt and pepper to taste. Adjust the spices if needed.

6. Remove the pot from the heat. Serve the vegan black bean chilli hot, garnished with fresh cilantro. Provide lime wedges on the side for squeezing over the chilli, if desired.

Nutrition Facts (per serving, based on four servings):

- Calories: 320
- Fat: 7g
- Carbohydrates: 55g
- Fibre: 16g
- Protein: 15g
- Sugar: 9g
- Sodium: 700mg

BUTTERNUT SQUASH AND KALE SALAD WITH MAPLE-BALSAMIC DRESSING

Preparation Time: 15 minutes Cooking Time: 25 minutes Serving: 4 servings

Ingredients:

- One small butternut squash, peeled, seeded, and cut into 1-inch cubes
- One tablespoon of olive oil
- Salt and pepper to taste
- 4 cups kale, stems removed and leaves thinly sliced
- 1/2 cup dried cranberries
- 1/4 cup toasted pumpkin seeds
- 1/4 cup crumbled feta cheese

For the Maple-Balsamic Dressing:

- Three tablespoons of balsamic vinegar
- Two tablespoons of maple syrup
- 1 tablespoon Dijon mustard
- One clove of garlic, minced
- 1/4 cup extra virgin olive oil
- Salt and pepper to taste

Directions:

1. Preheat the oven to 400°F (200°C).

2. Place the butternut squash cubes on a baking sheet. Drizzle with olive oil, season with salt and pepper, and toss to coat evenly. Roast in the preheated oven for 20-25 minutes or until the squash is tender and lightly browned. Set aside to cool.

3. In a large salad bowl, combine the sliced kale, dried cranberries, toasted pumpkin seeds, and crumbled feta cheese. Set aside.

4. In a small bowl, whisk together the balsamic vinegar, maple syrup, Dijon mustard, minced garlic, olive oil, salt, and pepper until well combined.

5. Add the cooled roasted butternut squash to the salad bowl with kale. Drizzle the maple-balsamic dressing over the salad and toss to coat all the ingredients evenly.

6. Allow the salad to sit for about 10 minutes to let the flavours meld together.

7. Serve the Butternut Squash and Kale Salad with Maple-Balsamic Dressing as a side dish or a light lunch.

Nutrition Facts (per serving): Calories: 220 Total Fat: 13g Saturated Fat: 3g Cholesterol: 8mg Sodium: 180mg Total Carbohydrate: 26g Dietary Fiber: 4g Sugar: 12g Protein: 4g

Note: The nutrition facts are approximate and may vary depending on the ingredients used.

GRILLED PORTOBELLO BURGER WITH AVOCADO AIOLI

Preparation Time: 15 minutes Cooking Time: 15 minutes Serving: 4 burgers

Ingredients:

- Four large Portobello mushroom caps
- Four burger buns
- One ripe avocado
- 1/4 cup mayonnaise
- One clove of garlic, minced
- One tablespoon of lemon juice
- 1 tablespoon olive oil
- Salt and pepper to taste
- Optional toppings: lettuce, tomato slices, red onion slices

Directions:

1. Preheat your grill to medium heat.

2. Prepare the Portobello mushrooms by removing the stems and gently brushing off any dirt. If desired, you can also remove the gills from the undersides of the mushrooms using a spoon.

3. In a small bowl, mash the avocado until smooth. Add the mayonnaise, minced garlic, lemon juice, olive oil, salt, and pepper. Mix well to combine and set aside.

4. Place the Portobello mushroom caps on the preheated grill, smooth side down. Cook for about 5-6 minutes or until the mushrooms start to soften and develop grill marks.

5. Flip the mushroom caps and continue grilling another 5-6 minutes or until they are tender and cooked through.

6. While the mushrooms are grilling, lightly toast the burger buns the grill or in a toaster.

7. Once the mushrooms are done, remove them from the grill and let them cool slightly.

8. Spread a generous amount of the avocado aioli on the bottom half of each burger bun.

9. Place a grilled Portobello mushroom cap on top of the aioli.

10. Add your desired toppings, such as lettuce, tomato slices, and red onion.

11. Top the burger with the other half of the bun.

12. Serve the Grilled Portobello Burger with Avocado Aioli immediately, and enjoy!

Nutrition Facts (per serving):

- Calories: 280
- Total Fat: 16g
- Saturated Fat: 2.5g
- Cholesterol: 5mg
- Sodium: 330mg
- Total Carbohydrate: 29g
- Dietary Fiber: 8g
- Sugars: 3g
- Protein: 8g

Note: The nutrition facts are approximate and may vary based on the specific ingredients used.

QUINOA AND VEGETABLE STIR-FRY

Preparation Time: 15 minutes Cooking Time: 20 minutes Serving: 4

Ingredients:

- 1 cup quinoa
- 2 cups water
- 2 tablespoons vegetable oil
- Three cloves garlic, minced
- One small onion, diced
- 1 bell pepper, thinly sliced
- Two carrots, thinly sliced
- One zucchini, thinly sliced
- 1 cup broccoli florets
- 1 cup snap peas
- Three tablespoons soy sauce
- One tablespoon of sesame oil
- One tablespoon of rice vinegar
- Salt and pepper to taste
- Optional toppings: chopped green onions, sesame seeds

Directions:

1. Rinse the quinoa under cold water and drain. In a medium-sized saucepan, bring the water to a boil. Add the quinoa, reduce the heat to low, cover, and simmer for about 15 minutes or until

the quinoa is cooked and the water is absorbed. Remove from heat and let it sit, covered, for 5 minutes. Fluff the quinoa with a fork and set aside.

2. heat the vegetable oil over medium-high heat in a large skillet or wok.

3. Add the bell pepper, carrots, zucchini, broccoli florets, and snap peas to the skillet. Stir-fry the vegetables for about 5-6 minutes until they are crisp-tender but retain their vibrant colours.

4. Mix the ingredients in a low-volume dish using a whisk. soy sauce, sesame oil, rice vinegar, salt, and pepper. Pour the sauce over the vegetables in the skillet and stir to coat evenly.

5. Add the cooked quinoa to the skillet Cook for an additional 2-3 minutes to heat the quinoa through.

6. Remove the stir-fry from the heat and serve hot. You can garnish it with chopped green onions and sesame seeds if desired.

Nutrition Facts (per serving):

- Calories: 285
- Fat: 9g
- Carbohydrates: 43g
- Fibre: 8g
- Protein: 9g

ROASTED BEET AND GOAT CHEESE SALAD

Preparation Time: 15 minutes Cooking Time: 45 minutes Serving: 4

Ingredients:

- Four medium-sized beets
- 4 cups mixed salad greens
- 4 ounces goat cheese, crumbled
- 1/2 cup walnuts, toasted and chopped
- Two tablespoons of balsamic vinegar
- Two tablespoons extra-virgin olive oil
- Salt and pepper to taste

Directions:

1. Preheat your oven to 400°F (200°C).

2. Trim off the beet greens and scrub the beets to remove dirt.

3. Place the beets on a baking sheet and drizzle them with olive oil. Season with salt and pepper.

4. Roast the beets in the preheated oven for about 45 minutes or until they are tender when pierced with a fork.

5. Once the beets are cooked, remove them from the oven and let them cool for a few minutes.

6. Once the beets are cool enough to handle, peel off the skins. They should come off quickly.

7. Cut the roasted beets into bite-sized wedges or slices.

8. In a large salad bowl, combine the mixed salad greens, roasted beet wedges, crumbled goat cheese, and toasted walnuts.

9. whisk the balsamic vinegar and extra-virgin olive oil in a small bowl. Season with salt and pepper to taste.

10. Drizzle the dressing over the salad and toss gently to coat all the ingredients.

11. Serve the roasted beet and goat cheese salad immediately.

Nutrition Facts (per serving):

- Calories: 250
- Total Fat: 18g
- Saturated Fat: 6g
- Cholesterol: 15mg
- Sodium: 220mg
- Carbohydrates: 15g
- Fibre: 4g
- Sugar: 9g
- Protein: 9g

Note: The nutrition facts are approximate and may vary based on the specific ingredients used.

SWEET POTATO AND CHICKPEA BUDDHA BOWL

Preparation Time: 15 minutes Cooking Time: 30 minutes Serving: 4

Ingredients:

- Two large sweet potatoes peeled and cut into cubes

- One can (15 ounces) of chickpeas, drained and rinsed
- One tablespoon of olive oil
- One teaspoon of ground cumin
- One teaspoon of smoked paprika
- 1/2 teaspoon garlic powder
- Salt and pepper to taste
- 4 cups cooked quinoa or rice
- 2 cups baby spinach or mixed greens
- 1/2 cup cherry tomatoes, halved
- 1/2 cup cucumber, diced
- 1/4 cup red onion, thinly sliced
- 1/4 cup fresh cilantro, chopped
- 1/4 cup unsalted roasted peanuts, chopped (optional)
- Lemon wedges for serving

Directions:

1. Preheat the oven to 425°F (220°C).

2. In a large bowl, combine the sweet potato cubes, chickpeas, olive oil, cumin, smoked paprika, garlic powder, salt, and pepper. Toss until the sweet potatoes and chickpeas are evenly coated with the spices.

3. Spread the sweet potato and chickpea mixture in a single layer on a baking sheet. Bake in the preheated oven for about 25-30 minutes or until the sweet potatoes are tender and golden brown.

4. While the sweet potatoes and chickpeas are roasting, prepare the remaining ingredients. Cook the quinoa or rice according to package instructions.

5. In serving bowls, divide the cooked quinoa or rice, baby spinach or mixed greens, cherry tomatoes, cucumber, and red onion.

6. Once the sweet potatoes and chickpeas are cooked, remove them from the oven and let them cool slightly.

7. Add the roasted sweet potatoes and chickpeas to the serving bowls.

8. Sprinkle with fresh cilantro and chopped peanuts (if using).

9. Serve the Sweet Potato and Chickpea Buddha Bowl with lemon wedges on the side for squeezing over the bowl.

10. Enjoy your nutritious and delicious Sweet Potato and Chickpea Buddha Bowl!

Nutrition Facts (per serving): Calories: 380 Total Fat: 8g Saturated Fat: 1g Cholesterol: 0mg Sodium: 280mg Total Carbohydrate: 64g Dietary Fiber: 10g Total Sugars: 7g Protein: 13g Vitamin D: 0mcg Calcium: 80mg Iron: 4mg Potassium: 800mg Note: Nutrition facts may vary depending on the specific ingredients and brands used.

BAKED GARLIC HERB TOFU

Preparation Time: 10 minutes Cooking Time: 25 minutes Serving: 4 servings

Ingredients:

- One block of firm tofu drained and pressed

- Three tablespoons soy sauce
- Two tablespoons of olive oil
- Three cloves of garlic, minced
- One tablespoon of dried mixed herbs (such as thyme, rosemary, and oregano)
- 1/2 teaspoon salt
- 1/4 teaspoon black pepper
- Fresh parsley, chopped (for garnish)

Directions:

1. Preheat the oven to 400°F (200°C) and line a baking sheet with parchment paper.
2. Cut the tofu into 1/2-inch thick slices and pat them dry with a paper towel.
3. In a small bowl, whisk together the soy sauce, olive oil, minced garlic, dried herbs, salt, and black pepper.
4. Place the tofu slices in a shallow dish and pour the marinade over them. Gently toss the tofu to coat each slice evenly.
5. Let the tofu marinate for about 10 minutes, flipping the slices halfway through to ensure even absorption of flavours.
6. Arrange the marinated tofu slices on the prepared baking sheet, leaving space between each slice.
7. Bake in the preheated oven for 20-25 minutes or until the tofu turns golden brown and slightly crispy on the edges.
8. Remove the baked tofu from the oven and allow it to cool for a few minutes.
9. Garnish with freshly chopped parsley before serving.
10. Serve the baked garlic herb tofu as a main dish or use it as a protein-rich addition to salads, stir-fries, or sandwiches.

Nutrition Facts (per serving):

- Calories: 180
- Total Fat: 12g
- Saturated Fat: 1.5g
- Cholesterol: 0mg
- Sodium: 620mg
- Carbohydrates: 5g
- Fibre: 2g
- Sugars: 1g
- Protein: 16g
- Vitamin D: 0mcg
- Calcium: 350mg
- Iron: 3mg
- Potassium: 360mg

Note: Nutrition facts are approximate and may vary depending on the specific brand of ingredients used.

STUFFED ACORN SQUASH WITH QUINOA AND CRANBERRIES

Preparation Time: 15 minutes Cooking Time: 1 hour Serving: 4 servings

Ingredients:

- 2 acorn squashes
- 1 cup quinoa, rinsed
- 2 cups vegetable broth
- One tablespoon of olive oil
- One small onion, finely chopped
- Two cloves garlic, minced
- One teaspoon of dried thyme
- 1/2 teaspoon ground cinnamon
- 1/2 cup dried cranberries
- 1/2 cup chopped pecans
- Salt and pepper to taste

Directions:

1. Preheat your oven to 375°F (190°C). Cut the acorn squashes in half lengthwise and scoop out the seeds and membranes. Place them cut side down on a baking sheet lined with parchment paper. Bake for about 30-35 minutes or until the flesh is tender.

2. While the squashes are baking, prepare the quinoa. In a medium saucepan, bring the vegetable broth to a boil. Add the rinsed quinoa, reduce the heat to low, cover, and simmer for 15-20 minutes or until all the liquid is absorbed and the quinoa is tender. Set aside.

3. heat the olive oil over medium heat in a large skillet. Add the chopped onion and minced garlic, and sauté until the onion is translucent and fragrant about 5 minutes. Stir in the dried thyme and ground cinnamon, and cook for another minute.

4. Remove the skillet from the heat and add the cooked quinoa, dried cranberries, and chopped pecans. Mix well to combine all the ingredients. Season with salt and pepper to taste.

5. Once the acorn squashes are done baking, remove them from the oven and carefully flip them over so the cut side faces up. Divide the quinoa stuffing evenly among the squash halves, pressing it down gently.

6. Return the stuffed squashes to the oven and bake for another 20-25 minutes or until the tops are golden brown and the squashes are completely tender.

7. Remove from the oven and let the stuffed squashes cool for a few minutes before serving. Enjoy!

Nutrition Facts (per serving):

- Calories: 300
- Total Fat: 10g
- Saturated Fat: 1.5g
- Cholesterol: 0mg
- Sodium: 450mg
- Carbohydrates: 50g
- Fibre: 8g
- Sugars: 12g
- Protein: 6g

Please note that the nutrition facts may vary depending on the specific brands of ingredients used and any modifications made to the recipe.

MEDITERRANEAN GRILLED EGGPLANT SALAD

Preparation Time: 15 minutes Cooking Time: 15 minutes Serving: 4 servings

Ingredients:

- Two medium-sized eggplants
- Two tablespoons extra-virgin olive oil
- Two cloves garlic, minced
- One red bell pepper, diced
- One yellow bell pepper, diced
- One small red onion, thinly sliced
- 1 cup cherry tomatoes, halved
- 1/4 cup Kalamata olives, pitted and halved
- 1/4 cup fresh parsley, chopped
- 1/4 cup fresh mint leaves, chopped
- 1/4 cup crumbled feta cheese
- Juice of 1 lemon
- Salt and pepper to taste

Directions:

1. Preheat the grill to medium-high heat.

2. Slice the eggplants into 1/2-inch thick rounds. Brush both sides of the eggplant slices with olive oil and season with salt and pepper.

3. Grill the eggplant slices for about 3-4 minutes on each side until they are tender and have nice grill marks. Remove from the grill and let them cool slightly.

4. Once cooled, cut the grilled eggplant slices into bite-sized pieces.

5. In a large bowl, combine the minced garlic, diced bell peppers, sliced red onion, cherry tomatoes, Kalamata olives, parsley, and mint leaves.

6. Add the grilled eggplant pieces to the bowl and gently toss to combine all the ingredients.

7. Drizzle the lemon juice over the salad and season with additional salt and pepper to taste. Toss again to coat everything evenly.

8. Sprinkle the crumbled feta cheese over the top of the salad.

9. Serve the Mediterranean Grilled Eggplant Salad immediately or refrigerate for a couple of hours to allow the flavours to meld together.

Nutrition Facts: Serving Size: 1 serving Calories: 170 Total Fat: 11g

- Saturated Fat: 2g
- Trans Fat: 0g Cholesterol: 6mg Sodium: 250mg Total Carbohydrate: 17g

- Dietary Fiber: 6g
- Sugars: 9g Protein: 4g Vitamin D: 0mcg Calcium: 80mg Iron: 1mg Potassium: 630mg

BROCCOLI AND MUSHROOM STIR-FRY

Preparation Time: 15 minutes Cooking Time: 10 minutes Servings: 4

Ingredients:

- 1 large head of broccoli
- 8 ounces mushrooms (such as cremini or button mushrooms), sliced
- Two tablespoons of vegetable oil
- Three cloves garlic, minced
- 1-inch piece of ginger, grated
- Two tablespoons of soy sauce
- One tablespoon of oyster sauce
- 1 teaspoon sesame oil
- 1/2 teaspoon red pepper flakes (optional)
- Salt and pepper to taste

Directions:

1. Cut the broccoli into small florets. Peel the stalk and cut it into thin slices.

2. Heat the vegetable oil in a large skillet or wok over medium-high heat.

3. Add the minced garlic and grated ginger to the skillet and sauté for about 1 minute until fragrant.

4. Add the sliced mushrooms to the skillet and cook for 3-4 minutes until they soften.

5. Add the broccoli florets and sliced stalk to the skillet. Stir-fry for 4-5 minutes until the broccoli is tender-crisp.

6. In a small bowl, whisk together the soy sauce, oyster sauce, sesame oil, and red pepper flakes (if using).

7. Pour the sauce over the vegetables in the skillet and toss to coat evenly. Cook for an additional 1-2 minutes to heat through.

8. Season with salt and pepper to taste.

9. Remove from heat and serve the Broccoli and Mushroom Stir-Fry hot as a side dish or over steamed rice or noodles.

Nutrition Facts (per serving):

- Calories: 120
- Fat: 7g
- Carbohydrates: 11g
- Fibre: 4g
- Protein: 6g

Note: Nutrition facts are approximate and may vary based on specific ingredients.

BAKED FALAFEL WITH TAHINI SAUCE

Preparation Time: 20 minutes Cooking Time: 25 minutes Serving: 4 servings

Ingredients: For the falafel:

- 1 ½ cups cooked chickpeas
- 1 small onion, roughly chopped
- Three cloves garlic, minced
- 1/4 cup fresh parsley, chopped
- 1/4 cup fresh cilantro, chopped
- One teaspoon of ground cumin
- One teaspoon of ground coriander
- 1/2 teaspoon baking powder
- Two tablespoons of all-purpose flour
- One tablespoon of lemon juice
- Salt and pepper to taste
- Olive oil for brushing

For the tahini sauce:

- 1/4 cup tahini paste
- Two tablespoons of lemon juice
- 2 tablespoons water
- One clove of garlic, minced
- Salt to taste

For serving:

- Pita bread or flatbread
- Fresh salad vegetables (lettuce, tomatoes, cucumbers, etc.)

Directions:

1. Preheat your oven to 375°F (190°C).

2. In a food processor, combine the chickpeas, onion, garlic, parsley, cilantro, cumin, coriander, baking powder, flour, lemon juice, salt, and pepper. Pulse the mixture until well combined but still slightly chunky. Avoid overprocessing.

3. Using your hands, shape the falafel mixture into small patties or balls about 1 ½ inches in diameter.

4. Place the falafel on a baking sheet lined with parchment paper. Brush each falafel with olive oil.

5. Bake the falafel in the preheated oven for 20-25 minutes or until golden brown and crispy on the outside.

6. While the falafel is baking, prepare the tahini sauce. In a small bowl, whisk together the tahini paste, lemon juice, water, minced garlic, and salt until smooth and creamy. Adjust the consistency by adding more water if necessary.

7. Once the falafel is ready, remove it from the oven and let it cool slightly.

8. Serve the baked falafel with pita bread or flatbread, fresh salad vegetables, and a drizzle of tahini sauce. You can also add toppings like sliced tomatoes, cucumbers, or pickles.

Nutrition Facts (per serving):

- Calories: 280
- Fat: 12g
- Saturated Fat: 1.5g
- Sodium: 320mg

- Carbohydrates: 34g
- Fibre: 8g
- Sugar: 3g
- Protein: 11g

Note: The nutrition facts may vary depending on the specific brands or variations of ingredients used.

SPINACH AND ARTICHOKE STUFFED MUSHROOMS

Preparation Time: 20 minutes Cooking Time: 25 minutes Serving: 4 servings

Ingredients: For the falafel:

- 1 ½ cups cooked chickpeas
- One small onion, roughly chopped
- Three cloves garlic, minced
- 1/4 cup fresh parsley, chopped
- 1/4 cup fresh cilantro, chopped
- One teaspoon of ground cumin
- One teaspoon of ground coriander
- 1/2 teaspoon baking powder
- Two tablespoons of all-purpose flour
- One tablespoon of lemon juice

- Salt and pepper to taste
- Olive oil for brushing

For the tahini sauce:

- 1/4 cup tahini paste
- 2 tablespoons lemon juice
- Two tablespoons water
- One clove of garlic, minced
- Salt to taste

For serving:

- Pita bread or flatbread
- Fresh salad vegetables (lettuce, tomatoes, cucumbers, etc.)

Directions:

1. Preheat your oven to 375°F (190°C).

2. In a food processor, combine the chickpeas, onion, garlic, parsley, cilantro, cumin, coriander, baking powder, flour, lemon juice, salt, and pepper. Pulse the mixture until well combined but still slightly chunky. Avoid overprocessing.

3. Using your hands, shape the falafel mixture into small patties or balls about 1 ½ inches in diameter.

4. Place the falafel on a baking sheet lined with parchment paper. Brush each falafel with olive oil.

5. Bake the falafel in the preheated oven for 20-25 minutes or until golden brown and crispy on the outside.

6. While the falafel is baking, prepare the tahini sauce. In a small bowl, whisk together the tahini paste, lemon juice, water, minced garlic, and salt until smooth and creamy. Adjust the consistency by adding more water if necessary.

7. Once the falafel is ready, remove it from the oven and let it cool slightly.

8. Serve the baked falafel with pita bread or flatbread, fresh salad vegetables, and a drizzle of tahini sauce. You can also add toppings like sliced tomatoes, cucumbers, or pickles.

Nutrition Facts (per serving):

- Calories: 280
- Fat: 12g
- Saturated Fat: 1.5g
- Sodium: 320mg
- Carbohydrates: 34g
- Fibre: 8g
- Sugar: 3g
- Protein: 11g

Note: The nutrition facts may vary depending on the specific brands or variations of ingredients used.

CAULIFLOWER AND CHICKPEA CURRY

Preparation Time: 15 minutes Cooking Time: 30 minutes Serving: 4

Ingredients:

- One large cauliflower, cut into florets
- One can (15 ounces) of chickpeas, drained and rinsed

- One onion, finely chopped
- Three cloves garlic, minced
- One tablespoon of fresh ginger, grated
- One tablespoon of curry powder
- One teaspoon of ground cumin
- One teaspoon of ground turmeric
- 1/2 teaspoon chilli powder (adjust according to your spice preference)
- One can (14 ounces) of diced tomatoes
- 1 can (13.5 ounces) of coconut milk
- Two tablespoons of vegetable oil
- Salt, to taste
- Fresh cilantro for garnish

Directions:

1. Heat vegetable oil in a large pot or Dutch oven over medium heat. Add the chopped onion and sauté until it becomes translucent, about 5 minutes.

2. Add minced garlic and grated ginger to the pot and cook for an additional 1-2 minutes, stirring constantly to prevent burning.

3. Add the curry powder, ground cumin, ground turmeric, and chilli powder to the pot. Stir well to coat the onions, garlic, and ginger with the spices. Cook for another minute to release the flavours.

4. Add the cauliflower florets and chickpeas to the pot. Stir to combine and coat them with the spice mixture.

5. Pour in the diced tomatoes with their juices and coconut milk. Stir well to combine all the ingredients. Season with salt to taste.

6. Bring the mixture to a boil, then reduce the heat to low. Cover the pot and simmer for about 20-25 minutes, or until the cauliflower is tender, stirring occasionally.

7. Remove the pot from the heat Once the cauliflower is cooked to your desired tenderness. Taste and adjust the seasoning if necessary.

8. Serve the cauliflower and chickpea curry over steamed rice or with naan bread. Garnish with fresh cilantro leaves.

Nutrition Facts (per serving):

- Calories: 290
- Total Fat: 15g
- Saturated Fat: 9g
- Cholesterol: 0mg
- Sodium: 460mg
- Total Carbohydrate: 30g
- Dietary Fiber: 9g
- Sugars: 9g
- Protein: 9g

Note: The nutrition facts provided are estimates and may vary depending on the specific ingredients and brands used.

TOMATO BASIL ZUCCHINI NOODLES

Preparation Time: 15 minutes Cooking Time: 10 minutes Serving: 4 servings

Ingredients:

- Four medium zucchini
- Two tablespoons of olive oil
- Three cloves garlic, minced
- 2 cups cherry tomatoes, halved
- 1/4 cup fresh basil leaves, chopped
- Salt and pepper to taste
- Grated Parmesan cheese (optional for serving)

Directions:

1. Spiralize the zucchini using a spiralizer to create zucchini noodles. If you don't have a spiralizer, you can use a julienne peeler or a knife to thinly slice the zucchini lengthwise into noodle-like strips. Set aside.

2. Heat the olive oil in a large skillet over medium heat. Add the minced garlic and sauté for about 1 minute until fragrant.

3. Add the cherry tomatoes to the skillet and cook for 5 minutes, stirring occasionally, until the tomatoes soften and release their juices.

4. Add the zucchini noodles to the skillet and toss them gently with the tomatoes. Cook for 3-4 minutes or until the zucchini noodles are tender but still slightly crisp. Avoid overcooking, as the noodles can become mushy.

5. Stir in the chopped basil leaves and season with salt and pepper to taste. Remove from heat.

6. Serve the tomato basil zucchini noodles hot, garnished with grated Parmesan cheese if desired.

Nutrition Facts (per serving):

- Calories: 120
- Total Fat: 8g
- Saturated Fat: 1g
- Sodium: 55mg
- Total Carbohydrate: 10g
- Dietary Fiber: 3g
- Sugars: 6g
- Protein: 3g

Note: Nutrition facts may vary depending on the specific ingredients used and any optional toppings or additions.

VEGAN LENTIL MEATBALLS WITH MARINARA SAUCE

Preparation Time: 15 minutes Cooking Time: 30 minutes Serving: 4 servings

Ingredients: For the Lentil Meatballs:

- 1 cup cooked lentils
- 1/2 cup breadcrumbs
- 1/4 cup finely chopped onion
- Two cloves garlic, minced

- Two tablespoons ground flaxseed mixed with six tablespoons water (flax egg)
- 1/4 cup nutritional yeast
- One teaspoon of dried oregano
- 1/2 teaspoon dried basil
- 1/2 teaspoon paprika
- Salt and pepper to taste

For the Marinara Sauce:

- 2 cups tomato sauce
- 1/4 cup tomato paste
- 1/4 cup water
- One small onion, finely chopped
- Two cloves garlic, minced
- One teaspoon of dried basil
- One teaspoon of dried oregano
- 1/2 teaspoon dried thyme
- Salt and pepper to taste

Directions:

1. In a large bowl, combine the cooked lentils, breadcrumbs, chopped onion, minced garlic, flax egg, nutritional yeast, dried oregano, dried basil, paprika, salt, and pepper. Mix well until all the ingredients are evenly combined.

2. Preheat the oven to 375°F (190°C). Line a baking sheet with parchment paper.

3. Shape the lentil mixture into small meatballs, about 1 to 1.5 inches in diameter, and place them on the prepared baking sheet.

4. Bake the lentil meatballs in the preheated oven for about 25-30 minutes or until they are firm and slightly browned.

5. While the lentil meatballs are baking, prepare the marinara sauce. In a medium saucepan, heat a little oil over medium heat. Add the chopped onion, minced garlic, and sauté until the onion is translucent and fragrant.

6. Add the tomato sauce, tomato paste, water, dried basil, dried oregano, dried thyme, salt, and pepper to the saucepan. Stir well to combine. Simmer the sauce on low heat for about 10-15 minutes, allowing the flavours to meld together.

7. Once the lentil meatballs are cooked, remove them from the oven and let them cool slightly.

8. Serve the lentil meatballs with a generous amount of marinara sauce. You can serve them over pasta, spaghetti squash, or crusty bread.

Nutrition Facts (per serving): Calories: 250 Total Fat: 3g Saturated Fat: 0.5g Cholesterol: 0mg Sodium: 500mg Total Carbohydrate: 45g Fiber: 12g Sugar: 8g Protein: 15g

Note: Nutrition facts may vary depending on the specific ingredients and brands used.

QUINOA AND BLACK BEAN STUFFED SWEET POTATOES

Preparation Time: 15 minutes Cooking Time: 1-hour Servings: 4

Ingredients:

- Four medium-sized sweet potatoes
- 1 cup quinoa, rinsed
- One can (15 ounces) of black beans, drained and rinsed
- One red bell pepper, diced
- 1/2 red onion, diced
- Two cloves garlic, minced
- One teaspoon of ground cumin
- One teaspoon of chilli powder
- 1/2 teaspoon paprika
- Salt and pepper, to taste
- One tablespoon of olive oil
- 1/4 cup chopped fresh cilantro
- Lime wedges for serving

Directions:

1. Preheat the oven to 400°F (200°C). Place the sweet potatoes on a baking sheet and pierce them with a fork. Bake for 45-50 minutes or until tender.

2. While the sweet potatoes are baking, cook the quinoa according to the package instructions. Set aside.

3. heat the olive oil over medium heat in a large skillet. Add the diced red bell pepper, red onion, and minced garlic. Sauté for 5 minutes or until the vegetables are tender.

4. Add the cooked quinoa and black beans to the skillet. Stir in the ground cumin, chilli powder, paprika, salt, and pepper. Cook for an additional 2-3 minutes until the flavours meld together.

5. Once the sweet potatoes are done baking, remove them from the oven. Cut them in half lengthwise, and gently fluff the insides with a fork. Spoon the quinoa and black bean mixture over the sweet potato halves.

6. Garnish with chopped fresh cilantro and squeeze fresh lime juice over the top. Serve hot, and enjoy!

Nutrition Facts (per serving):

- Calories: 400
- Fat: 6g
- Carbohydrates: 75g
- Fibre: 14g
- Protein: 13g
- Sodium: 380mg
- Potassium: 1100mg
- Vitamin A: 18400 IU
- Vitamin C: 66mg
- Calcium: 115mg
- Iron: 6mg

Note: Nutrition facts may vary depending on the size of the sweet potatoes and the brands of ingredients used.

KALE AND ROASTED VEGETABLE SALAD WITH LEMON-TAHINI DRESSING

Preparation Time: 15 minutes Cooking Time: 30 minutes Serving: 4

Ingredients:

- One bunch, kale, stems removed and leaves torn into bite-sized pieces
- One small sweet potato, peeled and cubed
- One red bell pepper, seeded and sliced
- One zucchini, sliced
- One yellow squash, sliced
- One small red onion, thinly sliced
- Two tablespoons of olive oil
- Salt and pepper to taste
- 1/4 cup tahini
- Juice of 1 lemon
- Two tablespoons water
- Two cloves garlic, minced
- One teaspoon honey
- Two tablespoons chopped fresh parsley

Directions:

1. Preheat the oven to 400°F (200°C).

2. On a large baking sheet, toss the sweet potato, bell pepper, zucchini, yellow squash, and red onion with olive oil. Season with salt and pepper.

3. Roast the vegetables in the preheated oven for 25-30 minutes or until they are tender and slightly caramelized. Remove from the oven and let them cool slightly.

4. Meanwhile, in a small bowl, whisk together tahini, lemon juice, water, minced garlic, honey, and a pinch of salt until smooth and creamy. If needed, add more water to achieve the desired consistency.

5. In a large salad bowl, add the torn kale leaves. Pour the lemon-tahini dressing over the kale and massage it into the leaves with your hands for a few minutes until the kale starts to soften and wilt.

6. Add the roasted vegetables to the bowl with the kale and toss to combine.

7. Sprinkle with chopped parsley and adjust the seasoning with salt and pepper if necessary.

8. Serve the kale and roasted vegetable salad immediately. It can be enjoyed as a light lunch or a side dish with grilled chicken or fish.

Nutrition Facts: (Per serving) Calories: 220 Total Fat: 15g Saturated Fat: 2g Cholesterol: 0mg Sodium: 80mg Total Carbohydrate: 20g Dietary Fiber: 4g Sugar: 6g Protein: 5g

Note: The nutrition facts are approximate and may vary depending on the ingredients used.

PORTOBELLO MUSHROOM FAJITAS

Preparation Time: 15 minutes Cooking Time: 20 minutes Serving: 4 servings

Ingredients:

- Four giant Portobello mushroom stems were removed and sliced
- One red bell pepper, sliced
- One yellow bell pepper, sliced
- One green bell pepper, sliced
- One medium-sized red onion, sliced
- Three cloves of garlic, minced
- Two tablespoons of olive oil
- Two tablespoons of fajita seasoning
- Juice of 1 lime
- Salt and pepper to taste
- Eight small flour tortillas
- Optional toppings: guacamole, salsa, sour cream, chopped cilantro

Directions:

1. In a large bowl, combine the sliced mushrooms, bell peppers, onion, minced garlic, olive oil, fajita seasoning, lime juice, salt, and pepper. Toss everything together until the vegetables are evenly coated with the seasoning mixture.

2. Heat a large skillet or grill pan over medium-high heat. Add the vegetable mixture to the pan and spread it out in a single layer. Cook for about 10-12 minutes, stirring occasionally, until the mushrooms and peppers are tender and slightly charred.

3. While the vegetables are cooking, warm the flour tortillas according to the package instructions.

4. Once the vegetables are cooked, remove the pan from heat. Taste and adjust the seasoning if needed.

5. Serve the Portobello mushroom fajitas by spooning the cooked vegetables onto warm tortillas. Add desired toppings such as guacamole, salsa, sour cream, and chopped cilantro.

6. Roll up the tortillas tightly and serve immediately. Enjoy your delicious Portobello mushroom fajitas!

Nutrition Facts (per serving):

- Calories: 250
- Total Fat: 10g
- Saturated Fat: 1.5g
- Cholesterol: 0mg
- Sodium: 450mg
- Total Carbohydrate: 35g
- Dietary Fiber: 7g
- Sugars: 7g
- Protein: 7g

Note: Nutrition facts may vary depending on the brands and quantities of ingredients used.

COCONUT CURRY TOFU STIR-FRY

Preparation Time: 15 minutes Cooking Time: 20 minutes Serving: 4 servings

Ingredients:

- 14 oz (400g) firm tofu, drained and cubed
- Two tablespoons of vegetable oil
- One onion, thinly sliced
- Two cloves garlic, minced
- One red bell pepper, sliced
- 1 cup broccoli florets
- 1 cup cauliflower florets
- One carrot, thinly sliced
- One can (13.5 oz/400ml) of coconut milk
- Two tablespoons of soy sauce
- One tablespoon of curry powder
- One teaspoon of turmeric powder
- One teaspoon of ginger paste
- Salt and pepper to taste
- Fresh cilantro for garnish
- Cooked rice or noodles (optional)

Directions:

1. Heat one tablespoon of vegetable oil in a large skillet or wok over medium-high heat. Add the tofu cubes and stir-fry for 5-6 minutes until golden brown. Remove the tofu from the skillet and set aside.

2. In the same skillet, add the remaining tablespoon of vegetable oil and sauté the onion and garlic until fragrant and translucent.

3. Add the red bell pepper, broccoli, cauliflower, and carrot to the skillet. Stir-fry for 3-4 minutes until the vegetables are slightly tender.

4. In a bowl, whisk together the coconut milk, soy sauce, curry powder, turmeric powder, ginger paste, salt, and pepper. Pour the mixture into the skillet with the vegetables.

5. Add the cooked tofu back into the skillet and stir everything together. Reduce the heat to medium-low and let the curry simmer for 10 minutes, allowing the flavours to meld together.

6. Taste and adjust the seasoning if needed. If you prefer a thicker sauce, you can simmer for a few more minutes until the desired consistency is reached.

7. Serve the Coconut Curry Tofu Stir-Fry over cooked rice or noodles if desired. Garnish with fresh cilantro.

Nutrition Facts (per serving):

- Calories: 280
- Fat: 21g
- Carbohydrates: 16g
- Protein: 11g
- Fibre: 4g

Note: The nutrition facts may vary depending on the specific brands and quantities of ingredients used.

MEDITERRANEAN QUINOA STUFFED TOMATOES

Preparation Time: 15 minutes Cooking Time: 30 minutes Serving: 4 servings

Ingredients:

- Four large tomatoes
- 1 cup cooked quinoa
- 1/2 cup diced cucumber
- 1/2 cup diced red bell pepper
- 1/4 cup chopped Kalamata olives
- 1/4 cup crumbled feta cheese
- Two tablespoons chopped fresh parsley
- Two tablespoons extra-virgin olive oil
- One tablespoon of lemon juice
- Two cloves garlic, minced
- Salt and pepper to taste

Directions:

1. Preheat the oven to 375°F (190°C). Slice off the tops of the tomatoes and scoop out the seeds and pulp using a spoon. Set aside.

2. In a mixing bowl, combine cooked quinoa, diced cucumber, red bell pepper, Kalamata olives, feta cheese, chopped parsley, olive oil, lemon juice, minced garlic, salt, and pepper. Mix well until all the ingredients are evenly distributed.

3. Stuff each tomato with the quinoa mixture, pressing it down gently to fill the tomatoes. Place the stuffed tomatoes in a baking dish.

4. Bake in the preheated oven for 25-30 minutes or until the tomatoes are soft and slightly wrinkled.

5. Remove from the oven and let the stuffed tomatoes cool for a few minutes before serving.

6. Garnish with additional chopped parsley if desired. Serve warm as a main dish or as a side dish to accompany a meal.

Nutrition Facts (per serving):

- Calories: 215
- Total Fat: 11g
- Saturated Fat: 3g
- Cholesterol: 8mg
- Sodium: 324mg
- Total Carbohydrate: 23g
- Dietary Fiber: 4g
- Sugars: 5g
- Protein: 6g
- Vitamin D: 0mcg
- Calcium: 86mg

- Iron: 2mg
- Potassium: 712mg

Note: The nutrition facts are approximate and may vary depending on the ingredients used.

BALSAMIC ROASTED VEGETABLES

Preparation Time: 15 minutes Cooking Time: 30 minutes Servings: 4

Ingredients:

- One medium-sized eggplant cut into 1-inch cubes
- Two zucchinis, sliced into 1/2-inch rounds
- One red bell pepper, seeded and sliced into strips
- One yellow bell pepper, seeded and sliced into strips
- One red onion, cut into wedges
- 8-10 cherry tomatoes
- Three tablespoons of balsamic vinegar
- Two tablespoons of olive oil
- Two cloves garlic, minced
- One teaspoon of dried thyme
- Salt and pepper to taste

- Fresh basil leaves for garnish

Directions:

1. Preheat your oven to 425°F (220°C).

2. In a large bowl, combine the balsamic vinegar, olive oil, minced garlic, dried thyme, salt, and pepper. Mix well.

3. Add all the prepared vegetables (eggplant, zucchini, bell peppers, red onion, and cherry tomatoes) to the bowl with the balsamic mixture. Toss the vegetables until they are well coated with the marinade.

4. Spread the vegetables in a single layer on a baking sheet lined with parchment paper or foil.

5. Roast the vegetables in the preheated oven for about 25-30 minutes or until they are tender and slightly caramelized. Stir once or twice during cooking to ensure even roasting.

6. Remove the roasted vegetables from the oven and transfer them to a serving dish.

7. Garnish with fresh basil leaves before serving.

Nutrition Facts (per serving):

- Calories: 140
- Total Fat: 7g
- Saturated Fat: 1g
- Cholesterol: 0mg
- Sodium: 40mg

- Total Carbohydrate: 18g
- Dietary Fiber: 6g
- Sugars: 10g
- Protein: 3g

Note: The nutrition facts provided are approximate and may vary based on the specific ingredients used.

VEGAN LENTIL SHEPHERD'S PIE

Preparation Time: 20 minutes Cooking Time: 40 minutes Serving: 6 servings

Ingredients: For the lentil filling:

- 1 cup green or brown lentils
- 3 cups vegetable broth
- One tablespoon of olive oil
- One onion, diced
- Two carrots diced
- Two celery stalks, diced
- Three cloves garlic, minced
- One teaspoon of dried thyme
- One teaspoon of dried rosemary
- One teaspoon paprika
- Salt and pepper to taste

- 1 cup frozen peas
- 1 cup corn kernels

For the mashed potato topping:

- 2 pounds potatoes, peeled and cubed
- 1/4 cup vegan butter
- 1/2 cup unsweetened plant-based milk
- Salt and pepper to taste

Directions:

1. Rinse the lentils under cold water and drain. In a saucepan, combine the lentils and vegetable broth. Bring to a boil, then reduce heat and simmer for about 20 minutes or until the lentils are tender. Drain any excess liquid and set aside.

2. Preheat the oven to 400°F (200°C).

3. heat the olive oil over medium heat in a large skillet. Add the diced onion, carrots, and celery. Sauté for about 5 minutes until the vegetables have softened.

4. Add the minced garlic, dried thyme, rosemary, paprika, salt, and pepper to the skillet. Cook for another 2 minutes.

5. Stir in the cooked lentils, frozen peas, and corn kernels. Cook for an additional 2 minutes to heat through. Remove from heat.

6. In a separate pot, boil the peeled and cubed potatoes until tender. Drain the potatoes and return them to the pot.

7. Add the vegan butter and plant-based milk to the pot with the potatoes. Mash until smooth and creamy. Season with salt and pepper to taste.

8. Transfer the lentil filling to a baking dish and spread it evenly. Top with the mashed potatoes, spreading them to cover the filling completely.

9. Place the dish in the preheated oven and bake for 20 minutes or until the mashed potato topping is golden and slightly crispy.

10. Remove from the oven and let it cool for a few minutes before serving.

Nutrition Facts (per serving):

- Calories: 320
- Fat: 8g
- Carbohydrates: 52g
- Fibre: 12g
- Protein: 10g

Enjoy your Vegan Lentil Shepherd's Pie!

ZUCCHINI NOODLES WITH WALNUT PESTO

Preparation Time: 15 minutes Cooking Time: 10 minutes Serving: 2

Ingredients:

- Four medium-sized zucchini
- 1 cup fresh basil leaves
- 1/2 cup walnuts
- Two cloves garlic, minced
- 1/4 cup grated Parmesan cheese
- 1/4 cup extra-virgin olive oil

- Salt and pepper to taste
- Optional toppings: cherry tomatoes, shaved Parmesan cheese

Directions:

1. Prepare the zucchini noodles by spiralizing the zucchini using a spiralizer. If you don't have a spiralizer, you can use a julienne peeler to create long, thin strips. Set aside.

2. In a food processor, combine the basil leaves, walnuts, minced garlic, and grated Parmesan cheese. Pulse until the ingredients are roughly chopped.

3. While the food processor is running, slowly drizzle in the olive oil until the mixture becomes smooth. Season with salt and pepper to taste. Set aside.

4. Heat a large non-stick skillet over medium heat. Add the zucchini noodles and cook for about 2-3 minutes, tossing them gently with tongs until they are slightly softened.

5. Remove the skillet from heat and add the walnut pesto to the zucchini noodles. Toss well to coat the noodles evenly.

6. Divide the zucchini noodles with walnut pesto into serving bowls. Top with cherry tomatoes and shaved Parmesan cheese, if desired.

7. Serve immediately and enjoy!

Nutrition Facts: (Note: The nutrition facts are approximate and may vary depending on the specific ingredients used.)

- Serving Size: 1/2 of the recipe
- Calories: 350
- Total Fat: 32g

- Saturated Fat: 5g
- Cholesterol: 7mg
- Sodium: 180mg
- Carbohydrates: 10g
- Fibre: 4g
- Sugar: 5g
- Protein: 8g

Please note that the nutrition facts provided are an estimate and can vary based on the specific ingredients and quantities used.

CHICKPEA AND VEGETABLE COCONUT CURRY

Preparation Time: 15 minutes Cooking Time: 30 minutes Serving: 4

Ingredients:

- Two tablespoons of vegetable oil
- One medium onion, chopped
- Three garlic cloves minced
- 1 tablespoon fresh ginger, grated
- One red bell pepper, sliced
- One small eggplant, diced
- One medium zucchini, diced
- 1 cup cauliflower florets
- One can (14 ounces) of chickpeas, drained and rinsed

- 1 can (14 ounces) of coconut milk
- Two tablespoons of curry powder
- 1 teaspoon ground cumin
- One teaspoon of ground coriander
- One teaspoon of turmeric powder
- Salt and pepper to taste
- Fresh cilantro leaves, chopped (for garnish)
- Cooked rice or naan bread (for serving)

Directions:

1. Heat the vegetable oil in a large pot or skillet over medium heat.

2. Add the chopped onion, minced garlic, and grated ginger. Sauté for about 3-4 minutes until the onion becomes translucent.

3. Add the sliced red bell pepper, diced eggplant, zucchini, and cauliflower florets to the pot. Cook for another 5 minutes, stirring occasionally.

4. Stir in the drained chickpeas, coconut milk, curry powder, ground cumin, ground coriander, turmeric powder, salt, and pepper. Mix well to combine.

5. Reduce the heat to low, cover the pot, and simmer for 20 minutes, or until the vegetables are tender and the flavours have melded together.

6. Taste and adjust the seasoning if needed.

7. Serve the Chickpea and Vegetable Coconut Curry over cooked rice or with naan bread.

8. Garnish with fresh cilantro leaves.

Nutrition Facts (per serving):

- Calories: 320
- Total Fat: 17g
- Saturated Fat: 12g
- Cholesterol: 0mg
- Sodium: 480mg
- Total Carbohydrate: 37g
- Dietary Fiber: 10g
- Sugars: 9g
- Protein: 9g

Note: The nutrition facts are approximate and may vary depending on the specific ingredients and brands used.

ROASTED BRUSSELS SPROUTS AND QUINOA SALAD

Preparation Time: 15 minutes Cooking Time: 25 minutes Serving: 4 servings

Ingredients:

- 1 pound Brussels sprouts, trimmed and halved
- 1 cup quinoa
- Two tablespoons of olive oil
- One teaspoon salt

- 1/2 teaspoon black pepper
- 1/2 teaspoon garlic powder
- 1/4 teaspoon paprika
- 1/4 cup dried cranberries
- 1/4 cup chopped walnuts
- 1/4 cup crumbled feta cheese

For the dressing:

- Two tablespoons of olive oil
- Two tablespoons of balsamic vinegar
- One tablespoon honey
- One tablespoon of Dijon mustard
- Salt and pepper to taste

Directions:

1. Preheat the oven to 400°F (200°C). Line a baking sheet with parchment paper.

2. In a medium saucepan, cook the quinoa according to package instructions. Once cooked, fluff with a fork and set aside.

3. In a large bowl, combine the Brussels sprouts, olive oil, salt, black pepper, garlic powder, and paprika. Toss until the Brussels sprouts are evenly coated.

4. Transfer the seasoned Brussels sprouts to the prepared baking sheet and spread them out in a single layer. Roast in the preheated oven for 20-25 minutes or until the Brussels sprouts are crispy and browned.

5. While the Brussels sprouts are roasting, prepare the dressing. In a small bowl, whisk together the olive oil, balsamic vinegar, honey, Dijon mustard, salt, and pepper until well combined.

6. In a large salad bowl, combine the cooked quinoa, roasted Brussels sprouts, dried cranberries, chopped walnuts, and crumbled feta cheese.

7. Drizzle the dressing over the salad and gently toss to coat all the ingredients evenly.

8. Serve the Roasted Brussels Sprouts and Quinoa Salad immediately as a main course or as a side dish.

Nutrition Facts (per serving):

- Calories: 325
- Total Fat: 18g
- Saturated Fat: 3.5g
- Cholesterol: 5mg
- Sodium: 600mg
- Total Carbohydrate: 35g
- Dietary Fiber: 7g
- Sugars: 9g
- Protein: 9g

Note: The nutrition facts provided are estimates and may vary depending on the specific ingredients used and the portion sizes.

GRILLED VEGETABLE SKEWERS WITH BALSAMIC GLAZE

Preparation Time: 20 minutes Cooking Time: 15 minutes Servings: 4

Ingredients:

- One red bell pepper
- One yellow bell pepper
- One zucchini
- One yellow squash
- One red onion
- Eight cherry tomatoes
- Eight button mushrooms
- Two tablespoons of olive oil
- Salt and pepper, to taste

Balsamic Glaze:

- 1/4 cup balsamic vinegar
- One tablespoon honey
- One clove of garlic, minced

Directions:

1. Preheat your grill to medium heat.

2. Prepare the vegetables by cutting the bell peppers, zucchini, yellow squash, and red onion into bite-sized pieces.

3. Thread the vegetables onto skewers, alternating between different vegetables to create colourful skewers. If using wooden skewers, soak them in water for about 15 minutes before threading the vegetables to prevent them from burning on the grill.

4. Drizzle the vegetable skewers with olive oil and season with salt and pepper.

5. In a small bowl, whisk the balsamic vinegar, honey, and minced garlic to make the balsamic glaze.

6. Place the vegetable skewers on the preheated grill and cook for about 10-15 minutes, turning occasionally, until the vegetables are tender and slightly charred.

7. During the last few minutes of grilling, brush the balsamic glaze onto the vegetable skewers, turning them to coat all sides. Reserve some glaze for serving.

8. Remove the skewers from the grill and transfer them to a serving platter.

9. Drizzle the remaining balsamic glaze over the grilled vegetable skewers for extra flavour.

10. Serve the Grilled Vegetable Skewers with Balsamic Glaze as a delicious and healthy side dish or as a vegetarian main course.

Nutrition Facts (per serving):

- Calories: 135
- Fat: 7g
- Carbohydrates: 16g
- Fibre: 4g
- Protein: 3g
- Sugar: 10g
- Sodium: 146mg

Note: Nutrition facts are approximate and may vary depending on the ingredients used.

BUTTERNUT SQUASH AND BLACK BEAN ENCHILADAS

Preparation Time: 30 minutes Cooking Time: 45 minutes Servings: 4

Ingredients:

- 2 cups butternut squash, peeled and diced
- One can of black beans, drained and rinsed
- One small onion, diced
- Two cloves garlic, minced
- One red bell pepper, diced
- 1 cup frozen corn kernels
- One teaspoon of ground cumin
- One teaspoon of chilli powder
- Salt and pepper to taste
- Eight small flour tortillas
- 2 cups enchilada sauce
- 1 cup shredded cheddar cheese
- Fresh cilantro for garnish (optional)

Directions:

1. Preheat the oven to 375°F (190°C).

2. In a large skillet, heat some oil over medium heat. Add the diced butternut squash and cook for about 5 minutes until slightly tender.

3. Add the onion, garlic, red bell pepper, and corn kernels to the skillet. Sauté for another 5 minutes until the vegetables are tender.

4. Stir in the black beans, cumin, chilli powder, salt, and pepper. Cook for an additional 2-3 minutes to allow the flavours to blend.

5. Warm the flour tortillas in the microwave for a few seconds to make them more pliable.

6. Pour about 1/2 cup of enchilada sauce into the bottom of a baking dish.

7. Spoon the vegetable and bean mixture onto each tortilla, roll them up, and place them seam-side down in the baking dish.

8. Pour the remaining enchilada sauce over the rolled tortillas, ensuring they are evenly coated.

9. Sprinkle the shredded cheddar cheese over the top.

10. Bake in the preheated oven for 25-30 minutes or until the cheese is melted and bubbly.

11. Remove from the oven and let it cool for a few minutes.

12. Garnish with fresh cilantro, if desired, and serve hot.

Nutrition Facts (per serving):

- Calories: 380
- Fat: 12g
- Carbohydrates: 56g
- Fibre: 12g
- Protein: 16g

Note: The nutrition facts may vary depending on the specific brands and quantities of ingredients used.

STUFFED BELL PEPPERS WITH QUINOA AND CHICKPEAS

Preparation Time: 20 minutes Cooking Time: 45 minutes Servings: 4

Ingredients:

- Four bell peppers (any colour)
- 1 cup cooked quinoa
- 1 cup cooked chickpeas
- One small onion, diced
- Two cloves garlic, minced
- One carrot, grated
- 1 cup spinach, chopped
- One teaspoon of dried oregano
- One teaspoon of dried basil
- 1/2 teaspoon paprika
- Salt and pepper to taste
- 1 cup tomato sauce
- 1/2 cup shredded mozzarella cheese (optional)
- Fresh parsley for garnish

Directions:

1. Preheat your oven to 375°F (190°C). Grease a baking dish and set aside.

2. Slice off the tops of the bell peppers and remove the seeds and membranes. Please place them in the prepared baking dish and set aside.

3. heat some olive oil over medium heat in a large skillet. Add the diced onion and minced garlic, and sauté until translucent and fragrant.

4. Add the grated carrot and chopped spinach to the skillet, and cook until the spinach wilts.

5. Stir in the cooked quinoa, chickpeas, dried oregano, dried basil, paprika, salt, and pepper. Cook for another 2-3 minutes to allow the flavours to blend.

6. Spoon the quinoa and chickpea mixture into the bell peppers, filling them to the top. Press down gently to pack the filling.

7. Pour the tomato sauce over the stuffed bell peppers, covering them evenly. If desired, sprinkle shredded mozzarella cheese on top.

8. Cover the baking dish with foil and bake in the preheated oven for 30-35 minutes or until the bell peppers are tender.

9. Remove the foil and continue baking for an additional 10 minutes or until the cheese is melted and bubbly (if using).

10. Once cooked, remove from the oven and let the stuffed bell peppers cool for a few minutes.

11. Garnish with fresh parsley before serving.

Nutrition Facts (per serving):

- Calories: 250

- Fat: 5g
- Carbohydrates: 40g
- Fibre: 10g
- Protein: 12g
- Vitamin A: 100% RDA
- Vitamin C: 250% RDA
- Calcium: 15% RDA
- Iron: 25% RDA

Note: Nutrition facts may vary depending on the specific ingredients and brands used.

LENTIL AND SWEET POTATO CURRY

Preparation Time: 15 minutes Cooking Time: 30 minutes Serving: 4 servings

Ingredients:

- One tablespoon of vegetable oil
- One onion, diced
- Three cloves garlic, minced
- One tablespoon of grated fresh ginger
- Two teaspoons of curry powder

- One teaspoon of ground cumin
- 1/2 teaspoon ground turmeric
- 1/4 teaspoon cayenne pepper (optional, adjust to taste)
- Two medium sweet potatoes, peeled and diced
- 1 cup red lentils
- 1 (14-ounce) can of coconut milk
- 2 cups vegetable broth
- Salt to taste
- Fresh cilantro, chopped (for garnish)
- Cooked rice or naan bread (for serving)

Directions:

1. Heat the vegetable oil in a large pot or Dutch oven over medium heat. Add the diced onion and sauté until softened, about 5 minutes.

2. Add the minced garlic and grated ginger to the pot, and cook for 1-2 minutes until fragrant.

3. Stir in the curry powder, cumin, turmeric, and cayenne pepper (if using), and cook for another minute to toast the spices.

4. Add the diced sweet potatoes, red lentils, coconut milk, and vegetable broth to the pot. Stir well to combine all the ingredients.

5. Bring the mixture to a boil, then reduce the heat to low and cover the pot. Simmer for about 20-25 minutes, or until the sweet potatoes and lentils are tender and cooked.

6. Season the curry with salt to taste, and adjust the seasoning if needed.

7. Serve the lentil and sweet potato curry with hot over, cooked rice or naan bread. Garnish with freshly chopped cilantro.

Nutrition Facts: (Note: The following nutrition facts are approximate and may vary depending on the specific ingredients used)

Serving Size: 1/4 of the recipe Calories: 350 Total Fat: 12g

- Saturated Fat: 9g
- Trans Fat: 0g Cholesterol: 0mg Sodium: 500mg Total Carbohydrate: 49g
- Dietary Fiber: 10g
- Sugars: 7g Protein: 12g

Please note that the nutrition facts provided are estimates and can vary depending on the specific brands and quantities of ingredients used.

CAULIFLOWER RICE STIR-FRY WITH TOFU

Preparation Time: 15 minutes Cooking Time: 20 minutes Serving: 4

Ingredients:

- One medium-sized cauliflower
- Two tablespoons of sesame oil
- 1 cup firm tofu, cubed

- 1 cup mixed vegetables (carrots, bell peppers, broccoli, etc.), chopped
- Three cloves garlic, minced
- Two tablespoons of soy sauce
- One tablespoon of rice vinegar
- One teaspoon of ginger, grated
- 1/4 teaspoon red pepper flakes (optional)
- Salt and pepper to taste
- Fresh cilantro or green onions for garnish (optional)

Directions:

1. Cut the cauliflower into florets and remove any green leaves. Place the florets in a food processor and pulse until they resemble rice-like grains. Set aside.

2. Heat one tablespoon of sesame oil in a large skillet or wok over medium-high heat. Add the tofu cubes and cook until they turn golden brown on all sides. Remove the tofu from the skillet and set it aside.

3. add another tablespoon of sesame oil and minced garlic in the same skillet. Sauté for about 1 minute until fragrant.

4. Add the chopped mixed vegetables to the skillet and stir-fry for about 5 minutes until they are slightly tender.

5. Push the vegetables to one side of the skillet and add the cauliflower rice to the other side. Stir-fry the cauliflower for about 3-4 minutes until it becomes tender but retains some texture.

6. In a small bowl, whisk together the soy sauce, rice vinegar, grated ginger, and red pepper flakes (if using). Pour the sauce over the cauliflower and vegetables into the skillet. Stir

everything together to ensure the flavours are evenly distributed.

7. Add the cooked tofu back to the skillet and mix it with the cauliflower rice and vegetables. Cook for another 2-3 minutes until everything is heated through.

8. Season with salt and pepper to taste.

9. Serve the cauliflower rice stir-fry hot, garnished with fresh cilantro or green onions if desired.

Nutrition Facts (per serving):

- Calories: 180
- Total Fat: 10g
- Saturated Fat: 1.5g
- Cholesterol: 0mg
- Sodium: 500mg
- Carbohydrates: 15g
- Fibre: 5g
- Sugar: 6g
- Protein: 12g
- Vitamin D: 0%
- Calcium: 10%
- Iron: 15%
- Potassium: 600mg

Note: The nutrition facts are approximate and may vary based on the specific ingredients used.

GREEK SALAD WITH TOFU FETA

Preparation Time: 15 minutes Cooking Time: 0 minutes Serving: 4

Ingredients: For the salad:

- 4 cups romaine lettuce, chopped
- 1 cup cucumber, diced
- 1 cup cherry tomatoes, halved
- 1/2 cup red onion, thinly sliced
- 1/4 cup Kalamata olives, pitted
- 1/4 cup fresh parsley, chopped
- Two tablespoons fresh dill chopped

For the tofu feta:

- 12 ounces firm tofu, drained and crumbled
- Two tablespoons of lemon juice
- One tablespoon of apple cider vinegar
- One tablespoon of extra virgin olive oil
- 1/2 teaspoon dried oregano
- 1/2 teaspoon garlic powder
- Salt and pepper to taste

For the dressing:

- Three tablespoons extra virgin olive oil
- Two tablespoons of red wine vinegar
- One teaspoon of Dijon mustard

- One clove of garlic, minced
- Salt and pepper to taste

Directions:

1. In a large bowl, combine the romaine lettuce, cucumber, cherry tomatoes, red onion, Kalamata olives, parsley, and dill. Toss gently to mix everything.

2. In a separate bowl, prepare the tofu feta. In a small bowl, together the lemon juice, apple cider vinegar, extra virgin olive oil, dried oregano, garlic powder, salt, and pepper. Add the crumbled tofu to the bowl and gently toss to coat it with the marinade. Set aside.

3. In another small bowl, prepare the dressing. Whisk together the extra virgin olive oil, red wine vinegar, Dijon mustard, minced garlic, salt, and pepper until well combined.

4. Add the tofu feta to the salad bowl and drizzle the dressing over the top. Toss gently to combine all the ingredients and coat them with the dressing.

5. Serve the Greek salad with tofu feta immediately, and enjoy!

Nutrition Facts: (Note: Nutritional values may vary depending on the specific brands of ingredients used and any modifications made to the recipe.)

Serving Size: 1/4 of the recipe

Calories: 230 Total Fat: 17g

- Saturated Fat: 2g
- Trans Fat: 0g Cholesterol: 0mg Sodium: 380mg Total Carbohydrate: 11g

- Dietary Fiber: 3g
- Sugars: 4g Protein: 10g

QUINOA AND KALE STUFFED MUSHROOMS

Preparation Time: 20 minutes Cooking Time: 25 minutes Serving: 4 servings

Ingredients:

- Eight large portobello mushrooms
- 1 cup cooked quinoa
- 1 cup chopped kale
- 1/2 cup diced onion
- Two cloves garlic, minced
- 1/4 cup grated Parmesan cheese (optional)
- Two tablespoons of olive oil
- One teaspoon of dried oregano
- 1/2 teaspoon salt
- 1/4 teaspoon black pepper

Directions:

1. Preheat the oven to 375°F (190°C). Line a baking sheet with parchment paper.

2. Remove the stems from the mushrooms and gently scrape out the gills with a spoon. Set aside.

3. In a large skillet, heat olive oil over medium heat. Add diced onion and minced garlic, and sauté until the onion becomes translucent, about 2-3 minutes.

4. Add chopped kale to the skillet and cook until it wilts about 3-4 minutes.

5. In a mixing bowl, combine the cooked quinoa, sautéed kale and onion mixture, Parmesan cheese (if using), dried oregano, salt, and black pepper. Mix well.

6. Spoon the quinoa and kale mixture into the mushroom caps, pressing it down lightly.

7. Place the stuffed mushrooms on the prepared baking sheet and bake in the preheated oven for 20-25 minutes or until the mushrooms are tender.

8. Remove from the oven and let them cool for a few minutes before serving.

Nutrition Facts (per serving):

- Calories: 170
- Total Fat: 7g
- Saturated Fat: 1g
- Cholesterol: 2mg
- Sodium: 335mg
- Total Carbohydrate: 21g
- Dietary Fiber: 4g
- Sugars: 3g
- Protein: 8g

Enjoy your delicious Quinoa and Kale Stuffed Mushrooms!

ROASTED VEGETABLE BUDDHA BOWL WITH TURMERIC TAHINI DRESSING

Preparation Time: 15 minutes Cooking Time: 30 minutes Serving: 4

Ingredients: For the Roasted Vegetables:

- 2 cups cauliflower florets
- 2 cups broccoli florets
- Two medium carrots, sliced
- One red bell pepper, sliced
- One yellow bell pepper, sliced
- One medium zucchini, sliced
- One tablespoon of olive oil
- One teaspoon paprika
- 1/2 teaspoon cumin
- Salt and pepper to taste

For the Turmeric Tahini Dressing:

- 1/4 cup tahini
- Two tablespoons of lemon juice
- One tablespoon of maple syrup
- One teaspoon of turmeric powder
- Two tablespoons water (adjust as needed)
- Salt to taste

For the Buddha Bowl:

- 4 cups cooked quinoa or brown rice
- 1 cup baby spinach leaves
- 1/4 cup sliced almonds
- Fresh cilantro or parsley for garnish (optional)

Directions:

1. Preheat the oven to 400°F (200°C).

2. In a large bowl, combine the cauliflower florets, broccoli florets, carrots, red bell pepper, yellow bell pepper, and zucchini. Drizzle with olive oil and sprinkle with paprika, cumin, salt, and pepper. Toss well to coat the vegetables evenly.

3. Spread the vegetables on a baking sheet lined with parchment paper. Roast in the preheated oven for about 25-30 minutes or until the vegetables are tender and slightly browned. Remove from the oven and set aside.

4. While the vegetables are roasted, prepare the turmeric tahini dressing. In a small bowl, whisk together the tahini, lemon juice, maple syrup, turmeric powder, water, and salt until smooth and well combined. Adjust the consistency by adding more water if needed. Set aside.

5. To assemble the Buddha bowls, divide the cooked quinoa or brown rice among four bowls. Top each bowl with roasted vegetables, baby spinach leaves, and sliced almonds.

6. Drizzle the turmeric tahini dressing over the Buddha bowls. Garnish with fresh cilantro or parsley if desired.

7. Serve the Roasted Vegetable Buddha Bowls immediately and enjoy!

Nutrition Facts (per serving):

- Calories: 350
- Total Fat: 15g
- Saturated Fat: 2g
- Sodium: 150mg
- Carbohydrates: 45g
- Fibre: 9g
- Sugar: 9g
- Protein: 11g
- Vitamin C: 100% DV
- Iron: 20% DV
- Calcium: 8% DV

Note: The nutrition facts are approximate and may vary based on the specific ingredients used.

PORTOBELLO MUSHROOM BURGERS WITH CARAMELIZED ONIONS

Preparation Time: 15 minutes Cooking Time: 25 minutes Serving: 4 burgers

Ingredients:

- Four large portobello mushrooms
- Two tablespoons of olive oil

- Two tablespoons of balsamic vinegar
- Four burger buns
- One large red onion, thinly sliced
- Two tablespoons butter
- Salt and pepper to taste
- Optional toppings: lettuce, tomato, cheese, avocado

Directions:

1. Preheat your grill or stovetop grill pan to medium heat.

2. Remove the stems from the portobello mushrooms and gently scrape out the gills using a spoon. This will create more space for the toppings.

3. whisk together olive oil and balsamic vinegar in a small bowl. Brush this mixture onto both sides of the portobello mushrooms.

4. Place the mushrooms on the grill or grill pan, gill side down. Cook for about 5-7 minutes per side or until they become tender. Remove from heat and set aside.

5. While the mushrooms are cooking, heat butter in a large skillet over medium heat. Add the sliced red onions and sauté for about 10-15 minutes, stirring occasionally, until they become soft and caramelized. Season with salt and pepper to taste.

6. Toast the burger buns on the grill or in a toaster until they are lightly golden.

7. To assemble the burgers, place a grilled portobello mushroom on the bottom half of each bun. Top with a generous amount of caramelized onions. Add any optional toppings you desire, such as lettuce, tomato, cheese, or avocado. Finally, place the top half of the bun on the burger.

8. Serve the Portobello Mushroom Burgers with Caramelized Onions immediately and enjoy!

Nutrition Facts: Here is the approximate nutritional information for one serving (without optional toppings):

Calories: 250 Total Fat: 12g

- Saturated Fat: 4g
- Trans Fat: 0g Cholesterol: 10mg Sodium: 200mg Total Carbohydrate: 30g
- Dietary Fiber: 5g
- Sugars: 8g Protein: 8g

Please note that the nutrition facts may vary depending on the specific brands and quantities of ingredients used.

COCONUT CURRY VEGETABLE NOODLES

Preparation Time: 15 minutes Cooking Time: 20 minutes Serving: 4 servings

Ingredients:

- 8 ounces of rice noodles
- One tablespoon of coconut oil
- One small onion, thinly sliced
- Two cloves garlic, minced

- One tablespoon ginger, grated
- One red bell pepper, thinly sliced
- One carrot, julienned
- 1 zucchini, julienned
- 1 cup broccoli florets
- 1 cup snap peas
- One can (14 ounces) of coconut milk
- Two tablespoons of soy sauce
- Two tablespoons of red curry paste
- One tablespoon of lime juice
- Fresh cilantro, chopped (for garnish)
- Crushed peanuts (for garnish)

Directions:

1. Cook the rice noodles according to the package instructions. Drain and set aside.
2. Heat the coconut oil in a large pan or wok over medium heat.
3. Add the onion, garlic, and ginger to the pan and sauté for 2-3 minutes until fragrant and the onion is translucent.
4. Add the red bell pepper, carrot, zucchini, broccoli, and snap peas to the pan. Stir-fry for about 5 minutes until the vegetables are tender-crisp.
5. In a separate bowl, whisk the coconut milk, soy sauce, red curry paste, and lime juice until well combined.
6. Pour the coconut milk mixture over the vegetables in the pan. Stir well to coat the vegetables in the curry sauce.

7. Add the cooked rice noodles to the pan and toss everything together until the noodles are evenly coated in the sauce and heated through.

8. Remove from heat and garnish with fresh cilantro and crushed peanuts.

9. Serve the Coconut Curry Vegetable Noodles hot, and enjoy!

Nutrition Facts (per serving):

- Calories: 315
- Fat: 18g
- Carbohydrates: 34g
- Fibre: 4g
- Protein: 7g
- Sugar: 5g
- Sodium: 625mg

Note: The nutrition facts are approximate and may vary depending on the specific ingredients and quantities used.

BAKED SWEET POTATO FALAFEL

Preparation Time: 20 minutes Cooking Time: 25 minutes Serving: 4 servings

Ingredients:

- Two medium sweet potatoes peeled and cubed
- One can (15 ounces) of chickpeas, drained and rinsed
- Three cloves garlic, minced
- One small onion, finely chopped
- 1/4 cup fresh cilantro, chopped
- 1/4 cup fresh parsley, chopped
- Two tablespoons of lemon juice
- Two teaspoons of ground cumin
- One teaspoon of ground coriander
- One teaspoon paprika
- 1/2 teaspoon salt
- 1/4 teaspoon black pepper
- 1/4 cup chickpea flour (or all-purpose flour)
- Olive oil for brushing

Directions:

1. Preheat the oven to 400°F (200°C). Line a baking sheet with parchment paper.

2. Place the cubed sweet potatoes in a microwave-safe bowl. Cover the bowl and microwave on high for 5 minutes or until the sweet potatoes are tender.

3. In a food processor, combine the cooked sweet potatoes, chickpeas, garlic, onion, cilantro, parsley, lemon juice, cumin, coriander, paprika, salt, and black pepper. Pulse until well combined but still slightly chunky.

4. Transfer the mixture to a mixing bowl and stir in the chickpea flour. Mix until the mixture holds together well.

5. Shape the mixture into small patties, about 1 1/2 inches in diameter, and place them on the prepared baking sheet.

6. Brush the falafel patties lightly with olive oil.

7. Bake in the preheated oven for 20-25 minutes, or until the falafel is golden brown and crispy, flipping them over halfway through cooking.

8. Remove from the oven and let the falafel cool for a few minutes before serving.

Nutrition Facts (per serving):

- Calories: 220
- Total Fat: 3g
- Saturated Fat: 0.5g
- Cholesterol: 0mg
- Sodium: 400mg
- Total Carbohydrate: 42g
- Dietary Fiber: 8g
- Sugars: 8g
- Protein: 8g

Note: Nutrition facts may vary depending on the specific ingredients and brands used.

MEDITERRANEAN ROASTED CAULIFLOWER SALAD

Preparation Time: 15 minutes Cooking Time: 30 minutes Serving: 4

Ingredients:

- One medium head of cauliflower, cut into florets
- Two tablespoons of olive oil
- One teaspoon of ground cumin
- One teaspoon of ground paprika
- Salt and black pepper to taste
- 1 cup cherry tomatoes, halved
- 1/2 cup Kalamata olives, pitted and halved
- 1/2 cup crumbled feta cheese
- 1/4 cup chopped fresh parsley
- 1/4 cup chopped fresh mint
- Juice of 1 lemon
- Two tablespoons extra-virgin olive oil

Directions:

1. Preheat your oven to 425°F (220°C).

2. In a large mixing bowl, combine the cauliflower florets, olive oil, ground cumin, paprika, salt, and black pepper. Toss well to coat the cauliflower evenly.

3. Spread the seasoned cauliflower on a baking sheet in a single layer. Roast in the preheated oven for about 25-30 minutes or

until the cauliflower is tender and golden brown, stirring once halfway through.

4. While the cauliflower is roasting, prepare the remaining ingredients. In a large serving bowl, combine the cherry tomatoes, Kalamata olives, crumbled feta cheese, chopped parsley, and chopped mint.

5. Once the cauliflower is done, remove it from the oven and let it cool for a few minutes.

6. Add the roasted cauliflower to the serving bowl with the other ingredients.

7. Drizzle the lemon juice and extra-virgin olive oil over the salad. Toss gently to combine all the ingredients and coat them with the dressing.

8. Taste and adjust the seasoning if needed with additional salt and pepper.

9. Serve the Mediterranean Roasted Cauliflower Salad at room temperature or chilled. It can be enjoyed as a side dish or a light main course.

Nutrition Facts: (Per serving) Calories: 210 Total Fat: 15g Saturated Fat: 4g Cholesterol: 15mg Sodium: 470mg Carbohydrates: 16g Fiber: 6g Sugar: 6g Protein: 7g

VEGAN LENTIL SLOPPY JOES

Preparation Time: 15 minutes Cooking Time: 35 minutes Serving: 4

Ingredients:

- 1 cup dry green lentils
- 2 cups vegetable broth
- One tablespoon of olive oil
- One small onion, diced
- Two cloves garlic, minced
- One red bell pepper, diced
- One carrot, grated
- One can (14 ounces) of crushed tomatoes
- Two tablespoons of tomato paste
- Two tablespoons maple syrup or agave nectar
- One tablespoon of soy sauce
- One tablespoon Worcestershire sauce (vegan if desired)
- One teaspoon of chilli powder
- 1/2 teaspoon smoked paprika
- Salt and pepper, to taste
- Four whole wheat burger buns

Directions:

1. Rinse the lentils under cold water and drain them.

2. bring the vegetable broth to a boil in a medium saucepan. Add the lentils, reduce the heat, cover, and simmer for about 20 minutes or until the lentils are tender. Drain any excess liquid and set aside.

3. heat the olive oil over medium heat in a large skillet.

4. Add the diced red bell pepper and grated carrot to the skillet. Cook for about 5 minutes, until the vegetables are tender.

5. Stir in the cooked lentils, crushed tomatoes, tomato paste, maple syrup or agave nectar, soy sauce, Worcestershire sauce, chilli powder, smoked paprika, salt, and pepper. Mix well to combine all the ingredients.

6. Reduce the heat to low and simmer the mixture for about 10 minutes, allowing the flavours to meld together. If the mixture seems too thick, add a little water or vegetable broth to thin it out.

7. Taste and adjust the seasonings if needed.

8. Toast the whole wheat burger buns, if desired.

9. To serve, spoon the lentil mixture onto the bottom half of each burger bun. Place the top half of the bun on top.

10. Vegan Lentil Sloppy Joes are ready to be enjoyed!

Nutrition Facts (per serving):

- Calories: 320
- Fat: 5g
- Carbohydrates: 58g
- Fibre: 12g
- Protein: 14g

Note: The nutrition facts may vary depending on the specific ingredients and brands used.

QUINOA AND BLACK BEAN SALAD WITH LIME-CILANTRO DRESSING

Preparation Time: 15 minutes Cooking Time: 20 minutes Serving: 4 servings

Ingredients: For the salad:

- 1 cup quinoa
- 2 cups water
- One can (15 oz) of black beans, rinsed and drained
- One red bell pepper, diced
- 1 cup cherry tomatoes, halved
- 1/2 cup diced red onion
- 1/2 cup chopped fresh cilantro
- One avocado, diced
- Salt and pepper to taste

For the dressing:

- 1/4 cup freshly squeezed lime juice
- Two tablespoons of olive oil
- Two tablespoons of honey or maple syrup
- Two cloves garlic, minced
- 1/4 cup chopped fresh cilantro
- Salt and pepper to taste

Directions:

1. Rinse the quinoa thoroughly under cold water. In a medium saucepan, bring the water to a boil. Add the quinoa, reduce heat

to low, cover, and simmer for 15-20 minutes, or until the water is absorbed and the quinoa is tender. Remove from heat and let it cool.

2. In a large bowl, combine the cooked quinoa, black beans, diced bell pepper, cherry tomatoes, red onion, chopped cilantro, and avocado.

3. In a small bowl, whisk together the lime juice, olive oil, honey (or maple syrup), minced garlic, chopped cilantro, salt, and pepper to make the dressing.

4. Pour the dressing over the quinoa and black bean mixture. Toss gently to combine and coat everything with the dressing. Adjust the salt and pepper according to your taste.

5. Serve the salad immediately or refrigerate for a couple of hours to let the flavours meld together.

Nutrition Facts (per serving):

- Calories: 320
- Total Fat: 12g
- Saturated Fat: 1.5g
- Sodium: 250mg
- Total Carbohydrate: 45g
- Dietary Fiber: 11g
- Sugars: 9g
- Protein: 10g
- Vitamin D: 0mcg
- Calcium: 50mg

- Iron: 3.5mg
- Potassium: 670mg

Enjoy your delicious and nutritious Quinoa and Black Bean Salad with Lime-Cilantro Dressing!

ZUCCHINI NOODLES WITH ROASTED RED PEPPER SAUCE

Preparation Time: 15 minutes Cooking Time: 25 minutes Serving: 4 servings

Ingredients:

- Four large zucchini
- Two red bell peppers
- Two tablespoons of olive oil
- One small onion, diced
- Two cloves garlic, minced
- One can (14 ounces) of diced tomatoes
- One teaspoon of dried oregano
- One teaspoon of dried basil
- 1/2 teaspoon salt
- 1/4 teaspoon black pepper
- 1/4 cup grated Parmesan cheese (optional)

- Fresh basil leaves for garnish

Directions:

1. Preheat your oven to 400°F (200°C). Line a baking sheet with parchment paper.

2. Cut the zucchini into long, thin strips resembling noodles using a spiralizer or a vegetable peeler. Set aside.

3. Place the red bell peppers on the prepared baking sheet and roast them in the preheated oven for about 20 minutes or until the skin is charred. Remove from the oven and let them cool for a few minutes.

4. Once the red bell peppers are cool enough to handle, remove the skin, seeds, and stems. Chop the peppers into small pieces and set aside.

5. heat the olive oil over medium heat in a large skillet. Add the diced onion and minced garlic, and sauté until they become translucent and fragrant.

6. Add the chopped roasted red peppers to the skillet, along with the diced tomatoes, dried oregano, dried basil, salt, and black pepper. Stir well to combine.

7. Reduce the heat to low and let the sauce simmer for about 10 minutes, allowing the flavours to meld together.

8. While the sauce is simmering, heat a separate skillet over medium heat. Add the zucchini noodles and cook for 2-3 minutes, tossing them gently until they are tender. Be careful not to overcook them, as they can become mushy.

9. Divide the zucchini noodles among four plates and top them with the roasted red pepper sauce.

10. If desired, sprinkle grated Parmesan cheese over the top and garnish with fresh basil leaves.

11. Serve the zucchini noodles with roasted red pepper sauce immediately.

Nutrition Facts (per serving):

- Calories: 120
- Fat: 6g
- Carbohydrates: 15g
- Fibre: 5g
- Protein: 4g
- Sugar: 9g
- Sodium: 450mg

Note: The nutrition facts are approximate and may vary depending on the ingredients used.

BUTTERNUT SQUASH AND LENTIL CURRY

Preparation Time: 15 minutes Cooking Time: 35 minutes Serving: 4 servings

Ingredients:

- One butternut squash, peeled, seeded, and cubed

- 1 cup red lentils
- One onion, diced
- Three cloves of garlic, minced
- 1-inch piece of fresh ginger, grated
- One tablespoon of curry powder
- One teaspoon of ground cumin
- One teaspoon of ground turmeric
- One can (14 ounces) of coconut milk
- One can (14 ounces) of diced tomatoes
- 2 cups vegetable broth
- One tablespoon of olive oil
- Salt and pepper to taste
- Fresh cilantro for garnish

Directions:

1. Heat olive oil in a large pot over medium heat. Add the diced onion and sauté until it becomes translucent, about 5 minutes. Stir in the minced garlic and grated ginger and cook for another minute.

2. Add the curry powder, cumin, and turmeric to the pot and stir well to coat the onion mixture with the spices. Cook for a minute to allow the flavours to develop.

3. Add the cubed butternut squash, red lentils, coconut milk, diced tomatoes (with their juices), and vegetable broth to the pot. Stir everything together and season with salt and pepper to taste.

4. Bring the mixture to a boil, then reduce the heat to low. Cover the pot and let it simmer for about 25-30 minutes, or until the butternut squash and lentils are tender and cooked through. Stir occasionally to prevent sticking.

5. Once the curry is cooked, taste and adjust the seasoning if needed. If you prefer a thinner consistency, add more vegetable broth or water.

6. Serve the butternut squash and lentil curry hot, garnished with fresh cilantro. It pairs well with steamed rice or naan bread.

Nutrition Facts (per serving):

- Calories: 280
- Fat: 9g
- Carbohydrates: 42g
- Fibre: 10g
- Protein: 10g
- Sodium: 480mg

Note: The nutrition facts are approximate and may vary based on the specific ingredients and quantities used.

CAULIFLOWER TABBOULEH

Preparation Time: 15 minutes Cooking Time: 0 minutes Serving: 4

Ingredients:

- One small head of cauliflower
- 2 cups fresh parsley, finely chopped
- 1 cup fresh mint leaves, finely chopped

- 1 cup cherry tomatoes, halved
- 1/2 cup cucumber, diced
- 1/4 cup red onion, finely chopped
- 1/4 cup extra-virgin olive oil
- Three tablespoons of lemon juice
- Salt and pepper to taste

Directions:

1. Wash the cauliflower head and remove the leaves and stem. Break the cauliflower into small florets.

2. Place the cauliflower florets in a food processor and pulse until they resemble rice-like grains. Alternatively, you can grate the cauliflower using a box grater.

3. Transfer the cauliflower "rice" to a large mixing bowl.

4. Add the chopped parsley, mint leaves, cherry tomatoes, cucumber, and red onion to the bowl with the cauliflower.

5. In a small bowl, whisk together the extra-virgin olive oil, lemon juice, salt, and pepper to make the dressing.

6. Pour the dressing over the cauliflower mixture and toss gently to combine all the ingredients.

7. Taste and adjust the seasoning if needed.

8. Allow the tabbouleh to sit for at least 10 minutes to allow the flavours to meld together.

9. Serve the cauliflower tabbouleh chilled as a side dish or refreshing salad.

Nutrition Facts (per serving):

- Calories: 120
- Total Fat: 9g
- Saturated Fat: 1g
- Sodium: 80mg
- Total Carbohydrate: 10g
- Dietary Fiber: 4g
- Sugars: 4g
- Protein: 3g

Note: Nutrition facts are approximate and may vary depending on the ingredients used.

ROASTED VEGETABLE AND QUINOA SALAD WITH LEMON-DIJON DRESSING

Preparation Time: 20 minutes Cooking Time: 30 minutes Serving: 4 servings

Ingredients:

- 1 cup quinoa
- 2 cups vegetable broth
- One red bell pepper, seeded and sliced

- One yellow bell pepper, seeded and sliced
- One zucchini, sliced
- One small red onion, sliced
- 1 cup cherry tomatoes
- Two tablespoons of olive oil
- Salt and pepper to taste
- 1/4 cup fresh parsley, chopped

For the Lemon-Dijon Dressing:

- Three tablespoons of lemon juice
- Two tablespoons of Dijon mustard
- One garlic clove, minced
- 1/4 cup olive oil
- Salt and pepper to taste

Directions:

1. Preheat the oven to 400°F (200°C).

2. Rinse the quinoa under cold water. In a saucepan, bring the vegetable broth to a boil. Add the quinoa, reduce the heat to low, cover, and simmer for about 15 minutes or until the quinoa is cooked and the liquid is absorbed. Remove from heat and let it cool.

3. On a large baking sheet, combine the red bell pepper, yellow bell pepper, zucchini, red onion, and cherry tomatoes. Drizzle with olive oil, season with salt and pepper, and toss to coat evenly.

4. Roast the vegetables in the preheated oven for 25-30 minutes or until they are tender and slightly charred, stirring halfway through. Remove from the oven and let them cool.

5. In a large bowl, combine the cooked quinoa, roasted vegetables, and fresh parsley.

6. In a small bowl, whisk together the lemon juice, Dijon mustard, minced garlic, olive oil, salt, and pepper to make the dressing.

7. Pour the Lemon-Dijon dressing over the quinoa and roasted vegetables. Toss gently to coat everything evenly.

8. Serve the Roasted Vegetable and Quinoa Salad with Lemon-Dijon Dressing as a main dish or a side dish. Enjoy!

Nutrition Facts (per serving):

- Calories: 320
- Fat: 18g
- Carbohydrates: 34g
- Fibre: 7g
- Protein: 8g
- Sugar: 7g
- Sodium: 450mg

Note: Nutrition facts may vary depending on the brands and quantities of ingredients used.

GRILLED EGGPLANT ROLL-UPS WITH CASHEW CHEESE

Preparation Time: 20 minutes Cooking Time: 15 minutes Servings: 4

Ingredients:

- Two large eggplants
- 1 cup raw cashews, soaked in water for 4 hours
- Two tablespoons of nutritional yeast
- Two cloves garlic, minced
- One tablespoon of lemon juice
- One teaspoon of dried basil
- One teaspoon of dried oregano
- Salt and pepper to taste
- 2 cups marinara sauce
- Fresh basil leaves for garnish

Directions:

1. Preheat your grill to medium-high heat.

2. Slice the eggplants lengthwise into thin strips, about 1/4-inch thick.

3. In a blender or food processor, combine the soaked cashews, nutritional yeast, minced garlic, lemon juice, dried basil, dried oregano, salt, and pepper. Blend until smooth and creamy. This is your cashew cheese filling.

4. Lay the eggplant slices on a baking sheet and brush both sides with olive oil.

5. Grill the eggplant slices for about 2-3 minutes per side or until they are slightly softened and have grill marks. Remove from the grill and let them cool slightly.

6. Spread a thin layer of the cashew cheese filling onto each eggplant slice.

7. Starting from one end, roll up the eggplant slice and secure it with a toothpick. Repeat with the remaining eggplant slices and filling.

8. In a baking dish, spread a thin layer of marinara sauce.

9. Place the eggplant roll-ups in the baking dish, seam-side down. Pour the remaining marinara sauce over the roll-ups.

10. Bake in a preheated oven at 375°F (190°C) for 15 minutes or until the sauce is bubbly and the roll-ups are heated.

11. Garnish with fresh basil leaves before serving.

Nutrition Facts (per serving):

- Calories: 250
- Total Fat: 12g
- Saturated Fat: 2g
- Sodium: 480mg
- Total Carbohydrate: 30g
- Dietary Fiber: 10g
- Sugars: 14g
- Protein: 9g

Enjoy your Grilled Eggplant Roll-Ups with Cashew Cheese!

SWEET POTATO AND LENTIL COCONUT CURRY

Preparation Time: 15 minutes Cooking Time: 35 minutes Serving: 4 servings

Ingredients:

- Two tablespoons of coconut oil
- One onion, diced
- Three cloves of garlic, minced
- One tablespoon of fresh ginger, grated
- Two sweet potatoes, peeled and cubed
- 1 cup red lentils, rinsed
- Two teaspoons of curry powder
- One teaspoon of ground cumin
- 1/2 teaspoon turmeric powder
- 1/4 teaspoon cayenne pepper (optional for spiciness)
- One can (14 ounces) of coconut milk
- One can (14 ounces) of diced tomatoes
- 2 cups vegetable broth
- Salt and pepper to taste
- Fresh cilantro, chopped (for garnish)

Directions:

1. Heat coconut oil in a large pot over medium heat. Add the diced onion and sauté until it becomes translucent, about 5 minutes.

2. Add the minced garlic and grated ginger to the pot, and cook for another minute, stirring frequently.

3. Stir in the sweet potatoes, lentils, curry powder, cumin, turmeric powder, and cayenne pepper (if using). Cook for 2-3 minutes to allow the spices to release their flavour.

4. Pour in the coconut milk, diced tomatoes, and vegetable broth. Stir well to combine all the ingredients. Bring the mixture to a boil.

5. Reduce the heat to low, cover the pot, and simmer for about 25-30 minutes or until the sweet potatoes and lentils are tender.

6. Season with salt and pepper to taste.

7. Serve the sweet potato and lentil coconut curry over cooked rice or with naan bread.

8. Garnish with fresh cilantro before serving.

Nutrition Facts (per serving):

- Calories: 350
- Fat: 15g
- Carbohydrates: 47g
- Fibre: 11g
- Protein: 9g
- Sugar: 9g

BROCCOLI AND CHICKPEA STIR-FRY

Preparation Time: 15 minutes Cooking Time: 15 minutes Serving: 4

Ingredients:

- One head of broccoli, cut into florets
- One can (15 ounces) of chickpeas, drained and rinsed
- One red bell pepper, sliced
- One medium onion, sliced
- Three cloves of garlic, minced
- Two tablespoons of soy sauce
- One tablespoon of sesame oil
- One tablespoon of vegetable oil
- One teaspoon of ginger, grated
- 1/2 teaspoon red pepper flakes (optional)
- Salt and pepper to taste
- Sesame seeds for garnish (optional)
- Cooked rice or noodles for serving

Directions:

1. heat the vegetable oil over medium-high heat in a large skillet or wok. Add the minced garlic, grated ginger, and red pepper flakes (if using). Sauté for about a minute until fragrant.

2. Add the sliced onion and red bell pepper to the skillet. Stir-fry for about 3-4 minutes until the vegetables start to soften.

3. Add the broccoli florets to the skillet and continue to stir-fry for another 3-4 minutes until the broccoli is bright green and slightly tender.

4. whisk together the soy sauce and sesame oil in a small bowl. Pour the mixture over the vegetables in the skillet. Stir to coat the vegetables evenly.

5. Add the chickpeas to the skillet and stir-fry for 2-3 minutes until heated through. Season with salt and pepper to taste.

6. Remove the skillet from the heat and serve the stir-fry over cooked rice or noodles. Garnish with sesame seeds, if desired.

Nutrition Facts (per serving):

- Calories: 240
- Fat: 8g
- Sodium: 550mg
- Carbohydrates: 34g
- Fibre: 9g
- Protein: 10g

STUFFED PORTOBELLO MUSHROOMS WITH QUINOA AND KALE

Preparation Time: 20 minutes Cooking Time: 25 minutes Serving: 4

Ingredients:

- Four large Portobello mushrooms
- 1 cup cooked quinoa
- 2 cups chopped kale
- One small onion, diced
- Two cloves garlic, minced
- 1/4 cup grated Parmesan cheese
- 2 tablespoons olive oil
- 1 tablespoon balsamic vinegar
- Salt and pepper to taste

Directions:

1. Preheat your oven to 375°F (190°C) and line a baking sheet with parchment paper.

2. Remove the stems from the Portobello mushrooms and gently scrape out the gills using a spoon. Set the mushrooms aside.

3. heat one tablespoon of olive oil over medium heat in a large skillet. Add the diced onion and minced garlic, and sauté until the onion becomes translucent.

4. Add the chopped kale to the skillet and cook until it wilts about 3-4 minutes. Season with salt and pepper to taste.

5. In a mixing bowl, combine the cooked quinoa with the sautéed kale mixture. Stir in the grated Parmesan cheese.

6. Place the Portobello mushrooms on the prepared baking sheet. Sprinkle them with salt and pepper and drizzle them with the balsamic vinegar and olive oil that is left over from cooking.

7. Fill each mushroom cap with the quinoa and kale mixture, pressing it down gently.

8. Bake the stuffed mushrooms in the preheated oven for about 20-25 minutes or until the mushrooms are tender and the filling is heated through.

9. Once cooked, remove the mushrooms from the oven

10. Serve the Stuffed Portobello Mushrooms with Quinoa and Kale as a main dish or as a side dish with your favourite salad or vegetable accompaniments.

Nutrition Facts (per serving):

- Calories: 225
- Total Fat: 10g
- Saturated Fat: 2g
- Cholesterol: 6mg
- Sodium: 180mg
- Total Carbohydrate: 28g
- Dietary Fiber: 5g
- Sugars: 4g
- Protein: 9g

QUINOA AND BLACK BEAN BUDDHA BOWL

Preparation Time: 15 minutes Cooking Time: 25 minutes Serving: 4 servings

Ingredients:

- 1 cup quinoa
- 2 cups water
- 1 can (15 oz) black beans, drained and rinsed
- 1 cup cherry tomatoes, halved
- One avocado, sliced
- 1 cup shredded carrots
- 1 cup cucumber, diced
- 1/4 cup chopped cilantro
- Two tablespoons of lime juice
- 2 tablespoons olive oil
- 1 teaspoon ground cumin
- Salt and pepper to taste

Directions:

1. In a medium saucepan, combine quinoa and water. Bring to a boil, then reduce heat to low, cover, and simmer for 15-20 minutes or until all the water is absorbed. Remove from heat and let it sit covered for 5 minutes. Fluff with a fork.

2. In a large bowl, combine the cooked quinoa, black beans, cherry tomatoes, avocado, shredded carrots, cucumber, and chopped cilantro.

3. In a small bowl, whisk together lime juice, olive oil, ground cumin, salt, and pepper. Pour the dressing over the quinoa mixture and toss gently to coat everything evenly.

4. Serve the Buddha bowl in individual bowls or plates, garnished with additional cilantro if desired.

Nutrition Facts (per serving):

- Calories: 380
- Total Fat: 17g
- Saturated Fat: 2.5g
- Cholesterol: 0mg
- Sodium: 220mg
- Total Carbohydrate: 48g
- Dietary Fiber: 12g
- Sugars: 4g
- Protein: 12g
- Vitamin D: 0mcg
- Calcium: 58mg
- Iron: 4mg
- Potassium: 745mg

ROASTED BRUSSELS SPROUTS AND FARRO SALAD WITH LEMON-TAHINI DRESSING

Preparation Time: 15 minutes Cooking Time: 25 minutes Serving: 4 servings

Ingredients:

- 1 pound Brussels sprouts, trimmed and halved
- 1 cup cooked farro
- 1/2 cup sliced almonds

- 1/4 cup dried cranberries
- Two tablespoons of olive oil
- Salt and pepper, to taste

For the Lemon-Tahini Dressing:

- 1/4 cup tahini
- Two tablespoons of fresh lemon juice
- One tablespoon honey
- Two tablespoons water
- Salt and pepper, to taste

Directions:

1. Preheat your oven to 400°F (200°C).
2. In a large mixing bowl, toss the Brussels sprouts with olive oil, salt, and pepper until evenly coated.
3. Spread the Brussels sprouts in a single layer on a baking sheet. Roast in the preheated oven for 20-25 minutes or until they become tender and lightly browned, stirring once halfway through cooking.
4. While the Brussels sprouts are roasting, prepare the Lemon-Tahini Dressing. In a small bowl, whisk together the tahini, lemon juice, honey, water, salt, and pepper until smooth. Set aside.
5. In a dry skillet over medium heat, toast the sliced almonds until golden brown and fragrant, frequently stirring to prevent burning. Remove from heat and set aside.
6. In a large salad bowl, combine the roasted Brussels sprouts, cooked farro, dried cranberries, and toasted almonds.
7. Drizzle the Lemon-Tahini Dressing over the salad and toss gently to coat all the ingredients evenly.

8. Taste and adjust the seasoning, if necessary, with salt and pepper.
9. Serve the Roasted Brussels Sprouts and Farro Salad immediately or refrigerate for later. It can be served warm or chilled.

Nutrition Facts (per serving):

- Calories: 300
- Fat: 18g
- Carbohydrates: 28g
- Fibre: 8g
- Protein: 10g

VEGAN LENTIL TACOS WITH AVOCADO CREMA

Preparation Time: 15 minutes Cooking Time: 30 minutes Serving: 4

Ingredients: For Lentil Filling:

- 1 cup dried lentils
- 2 cups vegetable broth
- 1 tablespoon olive oil
- One small onion, diced
- Two cloves garlic, minced
- One tablespoon of chilli powder

- One teaspoon of ground cumin
- 1/2 teaspoon paprika
- Salt and pepper to taste

For Avocado Crema:

- One ripe avocado
- 1/4 cup fresh cilantro, chopped
- Juice of 1 lime
- 2 tablespoons water
- Salt to taste

For Tacos:

- Eight small corn tortillas
- Shredded lettuce
- Diced tomatoes
- Sliced jalapenos (optional)
- Fresh cilantro for garnish

Directions:

1. Rinse the lentils under cold water and drain.

2. bring the vegetable broth to a boil in a medium-sized pot. Add the lentils and simmer for 20-25 minutes or until tender. Drain any excess liquid and set aside.

3. heat olive oil over medium heat in a large skillet. Add the diced onion and minced garlic, and sauté until the onion becomes translucent.

4. Add the cooked lentils, chilli powder, cumin, paprika, salt, and pepper to the skillet. Stir well to combine all the ingredients. Cook for an additional 5 minutes, allowing the flavours to meld together. Remove from heat and set aside.

5. To make the avocado crema, scoop the flesh into a blender or food processor. Add the chopped cilantro, lime juice, water, and salt. Blend until smooth and creamy. Adjust the seasoning to taste.

6. Warm the corn tortillas in a dry skillet or over an open flame until pliable.

7. To assemble the tacos, spoon the lentil filling onto each tortilla. Top with shredded lettuce, diced tomatoes, sliced jalapenos (if desired), and a drizzle of avocado crema. Garnish with fresh cilantro.

8. Serve the Vegan Lentil Tacos with Avocado Crema immediately, and enjoy!

Nutrition Facts (per serving): Calories: 250 Total Fat: 8g Saturated Fat: 1g Sodium: 200mg Carbohydrates: 38g Fiber: 12g Sugar: 2g Protein: 12g

ZUCCHINI NOODLES WITH CREAMY AVOCADO SAUCE

Preparation Time: 15 minutes Cooking Time: 0 minutes Serving: 2 servings

Ingredients:

- Two medium-sized zucchini
- 1 ripe avocado

- 1/4 cup fresh basil leaves
- Two tablespoons of lemon juice
- Two tablespoons of olive oil
- Two cloves garlic, minced
- Salt and pepper to taste
- Optional toppings: cherry tomatoes, grated Parmesan cheese, chopped parsley

Directions:

1. Wash the zucchini and trim off the ends. Using a spiralizer or vegetable peeler, create long, thin noodles from the zucchini. Set aside.

2. In a blender or food processor, combine the avocado, basil leaves, lemon juice, olive oil, minced garlic, salt, and pepper. Blend until smooth and creamy. If needed, add a little water to thin out the sauce.

3. In a large mixing bowl, toss the zucchini noodles with the creamy avocado sauce until well coated.

4. Serve the zucchini noodles in bowls and garnish with your preferred toppings, such as cherry tomatoes, grated Parmesan cheese, and chopped parsley.

5. Enjoy immediately as a refreshing and healthy meal!

Nutrition Facts (per serving):

- Calories: 180
- Total Fat: 15g
- Saturated Fat: 2g
- Sodium: 10mg

- Carbohydrates: 12g
- Fibre: 7g
- Sugar: 4g
- Protein: 4g
- Vitamin C: 30% DV
- Iron: 6% DV

Please note that the nutrition facts are approximate and may vary depending on the specific ingredients and quantities used.

MOROCCAN CHICKPEA STEW

Preparation Time: 15 minutes Cooking Time: 40 minutes Serving: 4 servings

Ingredients:

- Two tablespoons of olive oil
- One onion, diced
- Three cloves garlic, minced
- Two carrots, peeled and chopped
- Two bell peppers (red and/or yellow), chopped
- One teaspoon of ground cumin
- One teaspoon of ground coriander
- One teaspoon paprika
- 1/2 teaspoon ground cinnamon
- 1/4 teaspoon cayenne pepper (optional for heat)

- One can (14 ounces) of diced tomatoes
- One can (14 ounces) of chickpeas, drained and rinsed
- 1 cup vegetable broth
- 1 cup chopped kale or spinach
- Salt and pepper to taste
- Fresh cilantro or parsley, chopped (for garnish)
- Lemon wedges (for serving)

Directions:

1. Heat the olive oil in a large pot over medium heat. Add the onion and garlic and sauté until the onion is translucent and fragrant.

2. Add the carrots and bell peppers to the pot and cook for about 5 minutes until they soften.

3. Stir in the ground cumin, coriander, paprika, ground cinnamon, and cayenne pepper (if using). Cook for another minute to toast the spices and enhance their flavours.

4. Add the diced tomatoes, chickpeas, and vegetable broth to the pot. Bring to a simmer and let it cook for about 20 minutes, allowing the flavours to meld together.

5. Stir in the chopped kale or spinach and cook for another 5 minutes until the greens have wilted.

6. Season with salt and pepper to taste.

7. Serve the Moroccan Chickpea Stew in bowls, garnished with fresh cilantro or parsley. Squeeze some lemon juice over each serving for an extra tangy flavour.

Nutrition Facts (per serving):

- Calories: 250
- Total Fat: 7g
- Saturated Fat: 1g
- Cholesterol: 0mg
- Sodium: 600mg
- Total Carbohydrate: 40g
- Dietary Fiber: 10g
- Sugars: 10g
- Protein: 10g

Enjoy your delicious Moroccan Chickpea Stew!

GRILLED PORTOBELLO MUSHROOM STEAKS

Preparation Time: 15 minutes Cooking Time: 10 minutes Serving: 4 servings

Ingredients:

- Four large Portobello mushrooms
- Three tablespoons of balsamic vinegar
- Three tablespoons olive oil
- Two cloves garlic, minced
- One teaspoon of dried thyme
- Salt and pepper to taste

- Four slices of your favourite cheese (optional)
- Fresh parsley or basil for garnish (optional)

Directions:

1. Preheat the grill to medium-high heat.
2. Clean the Portobello mushrooms by gently wiping them with a damp cloth to remove any dirt. Remove the stems and set aside.
3. In a small bowl, whisk together balsamic vinegar, olive oil, minced garlic, dried thyme, salt, and pepper.
4. Brush both sides of the Portobello mushrooms with the balsamic mixture, ensuring they are well coated.
5. Place the mushrooms on the preheated grill, gill side down. Cook for about 5 minutes, then flip them over.
6. If desired, place a slice of cheese on top of each mushroom during the last 2 minutes of grilling to allow it to melt.
7. Remove the grilled mushrooms from the heat and transfer them to a serving platter. Sprinkle with fresh parsley or basil for added flavour and garnish.
8. Serve the Grilled Portobello Mushroom Steaks hot as a main dish or as a flavorful addition to salads, sandwiches, or wraps.

Nutrition Facts (per serving):

- Calories: 90
- Total Fat: 7g
- Saturated Fat: 1g
- Cholesterol: 0mg
- Sodium: 50mg

- Carbohydrates: 6g
- Fibre: 1g
- Sugar: 3g
- Protein: 3g

QUINOA AND VEGETABLE SUSHI ROLLS

Preparation Time: 30 minutes Cooking Time: 15 minutes Serving: 4 rolls (16 pieces)

Ingredients:

- 1 cup quinoa
- 2 cups water
- Four nori seaweed sheets
- One carrot cut into matchsticks
- One cucumber cut into matchsticks
- One red bell pepper cut into matchsticks
- One avocado, sliced
- Soy sauce for serving
- Pickled ginger for serving
- Wasabi, for serving

Directions:

1. Rinse the quinoa thoroughly under cold water. In a saucepan, combine the rinsed quinoa and water. Bring to a boil, then reduce the heat and simmer for 15 minutes or until the water is absorbed. Remove from heat and let it cool.

2. Place a bamboo sushi mat on a clean surface. Lay a sheet of nori on the mat.

3. Wet your hands with water to prevent sticking, then spread a thin layer of cooked quinoa evenly over the nori sheet, leaving about 1 inch of space at the top.

4. Arrange the carrot, cucumber, bell pepper, and avocado slices in a straight line across the quinoa, about 1 inch from the bottom of the nori sheet.

5. Using the bamboo mat, roll the nori tightly, starting from the bottom and applying gentle pressure. Wet the top edge of the nori sheet with a bit of water to seal the roll.

6. Repeat the process with the remaining nori sheets and ingredients.

7. Using a sharp knife, slice each roll into bite-sized pieces, about 1 inch thick.

8. Serve the sushi rolls with soy sauce, pickled ginger, and wasabi on the side.

Nutrition Facts (per serving):

- Calories: 280
- Total Fat: 9g
- Saturated Fat: 1g
- Cholesterol: 0mg
- Sodium: 400mg
- Total Carbohydrate: 45g
- Dietary Fiber: 9g
- Sugars: 4g
- Protein: 10g

CAULIFLOWER ALFREDO PASTA

Preparation Time: 15 minutes Cooking Time: 25 minutes Serving: 4 servings

Ingredients:

- One medium-sized cauliflower head cut into florets
- 8 ounces (225 grams) of fettuccine pasta
- Two tablespoons of olive oil
- Three cloves garlic, minced
- 1 cup vegetable broth
- 1 cup unsweetened almond milk (or any non-dairy milk)
- 1/2 cup nutritional yeast
- 1/4 cup fresh lemon juice
- Salt and pepper to taste
- Chopped fresh parsley for garnish (optional)

Directions:

1. In a large pot of salted boiling water, cook the fettuccine pasta according to the package instructions until al dente. Drain and set aside.

2. Meanwhile, steam the cauliflower florets until tender. This can be done by placing them in a steamer basket over boiling water for about 10-12 minutes or until easily pierced with a fork. Remove from heat and set aside.

3. heat the olive oil over medium heat in a large skillet. Add the minced garlic and sauté for 1-2 minutes until fragrant and lightly golden.

4. Transfer the steamed cauliflower florets to a blender or food processor. Add the sautéed garlic, vegetable broth, almond milk,

nutritional yeast, lemon juice, salt, and pepper. Blend until smooth and creamy, adjusting the seasonings to taste.

5. Return the cauliflower Alfredo sauce to the skillet and heat over low heat for 2-3 minutes, stirring occasionally, until heated through.

6. Add the cooked fettuccine pasta to the skillet with the cauliflower Alfredo sauce. Toss well until the pasta is evenly coated with the sauce.

7. Serve the cauliflower Alfredo pasta in individual bowls or plates. Garnish with chopped fresh parsley, if desired.

Nutrition Facts (per serving):

- Calories: 320
- Total Fat: 10g
- Saturated Fat: 1.5g
- Cholesterol: 0mg
- Sodium: 240mg
- Total Carbohydrate: 50g
- Dietary Fiber: 7g
- Sugars: 5g
- Protein: 12g

LENTIL AND SWEET POTATO TACOS

Preparation Time: 15 minutes Cooking Time: 30 minutes Serving: 4 servings

Ingredients:

- 1 cup dried lentils
- Two medium sweet potatoes, peeled and diced
- One small onion, finely chopped
- Two cloves garlic, minced
- One tablespoon of olive oil
- One teaspoon of ground cumin
- One teaspoon of chilli powder
- 1/2 teaspoon paprika
- 1/2 teaspoon salt
- 1/4 teaspoon black pepper
- 1/4 teaspoon cayenne pepper (optional, for extra heat)
- Eight small flour tortillas
- Toppings: diced avocado, chopped cilantro, salsa, lime wedges

Directions:

1. Rinse the lentils under cold water and drain them. In a medium saucepan, bring 3 cups of water to a boil. Add the lentils, reduce the heat to low, cover, and simmer for about 20 minutes or until the lentils are tender. Drain any excess water and set the cooked lentils aside.

2. Meanwhile, heat the olive oil over medium heat in a large skillet. Add the chopped onion, minced garlic, and sauté for about 5 minutes until they become translucent and fragrant.

3. Add the diced sweet potatoes to the skillet and season with cumin, chilli powder, paprika, salt, black pepper, and cayenne

pepper (if using). Stir well to coat the sweet potatoes with the spices.

4. Cover the skillet and cook for about 15 minutes, stirring occasionally, until the sweet potatoes are tender and slightly caramelized.

5. Add the cooked lentils to the skillet and stir everything together. Cook for an additional 3-5 minutes to allow the flavours to meld.

6. Warm the flour tortillas in a separate skillet or oven.

7. To assemble the tacos, spoon the lentil and sweet potato mixture onto each tortilla. Top with diced avocado, chopped cilantro, salsa, and a squeeze of lime juice.

8. Serve the Lentil and Sweet Potato Tacos immediately, and enjoy!

Nutrition Facts (per serving):

- Calories: 350
- Total Fat: 7g
- Saturated Fat: 1g
- Cholesterol: 0mg
- Sodium: 550mg
- Total Carbohydrate: 60g
- Dietary Fiber: 14g
- Sugars: 7g
- Protein: 12g

ROASTED VEGETABLE AND QUINOA BUDDHA BOWL

Preparation Time: 15 minutes Cooking Time: 30 minutes Serving: 4 servings

Ingredients:

- 1 cup quinoa
- 2 cups water
- One red bell pepper, sliced
- 1 yellow bell pepper, sliced
- One zucchini, sliced
- One small eggplant, diced
- One red onion, sliced
- Two tablespoons of olive oil
- One teaspoon paprika
- One teaspoon of garlic powder
- 1/2 teaspoon salt
- 1/4 teaspoon black pepper
- 4 cups mixed salad greens
- 1/4 cup chopped fresh cilantro
- 1/4 cup crumbled feta cheese (optional)
- 1/4 cup sliced almonds

For the dressing:

- Three tablespoons olive oil
- Two tablespoons of lemon juice
- One tablespoon honey
- One clove of garlic, minced

- Salt and pepper to taste

Directions:

1. Preheat the oven to 425°F (220°C).

2. Rinse the quinoa under cold water. In a medium saucepan, bring the water to a boil. Add the quinoa, reduce heat to low, cover, and simmer for 15-20 minutes or until the water is absorbed and the quinoa is cooked. Fluff with a fork and set aside.

3. On a large baking sheet, toss the bell peppers, zucchini, eggplant, and red onion with olive oil, paprika, garlic powder, salt, and black pepper. Spread the vegetables in a single layer and roast in the preheated oven for 25-30 minutes or until they are tender and slightly browned.

4. While the vegetables are roasted, prepare the dressing by whisking together olive oil, lemon juice, honey, minced garlic, salt, and pepper in a small bowl. Set aside.

5. Once the vegetables are done, assemble the Buddha bowls. Divide the cooked quinoa, roasted vegetables, mixed salad greens, cilantro, feta cheese (if using), and sliced almonds among four bowls.

6. Drizzle each bowl with the prepared dressing.

7. Serve the Roasted Vegetable and Quinoa Buddha Bowls immediately and enjoy!

Nutrition Facts (per serving):

- Calories: 385
- Fat: 21g
- Saturated Fat: 3g
- Cholesterol: 6mg

- Sodium: 352mg
- Carbohydrates: 44g
- Fibre: 8g
- Sugar: 9g
- Protein: 9g
- Vitamin D: 0mcg
- Calcium: 93mg
- Iron: 3mg
- Potassium: 680mg

MEDITERRANEAN BAKED EGGPLANT WITH TOMATO SAUCE

Preparation Time: 15 minutes Cooking Time: 40 minutes Serving: 4 servings

Ingredients:

- Two large eggplants
- Two tablespoons of olive oil
- One onion, finely chopped
- 3 cloves garlic, minced
- One can (400 grams) of crushed tomatoes
- One teaspoon of dried oregano
- One teaspoon of dried basil
- Salt and pepper to taste

- 1/2 cup grated Parmesan cheese
- Fresh basil leaves for garnish

Directions:

1. Preheat the oven to 375°F (190°C).

2. Slice the eggplants lengthwise into 1/4-inch thick slices.

3. Place the eggplant slices on a baking sheet and brush both sides with olive oil. Bake in the preheated oven for 10 minutes or until tender.

4. Meanwhile, heat one tablespoon of olive oil in a large skillet over medium heat. Add the chopped onion and minced garlic, and cook until the onion becomes translucent and the garlic is fragrant.

5. Stir in the crushed tomatoes, dried oregano, dried basil, salt, and pepper. Simmer the sauce for about 10 minutes, allowing the flavours to blend.

6. Remove the eggplant slices from the oven and spoon a small amount of the tomato sauce onto each slice. Roll up the slices and place them seam-side down in a baking dish.

7. Pour the remaining tomato sauce over the rolled eggplant slices, and sprinkle the grated Parmesan cheese on top.

8. Bake the dish in the oven for 20 minutes or until the cheese is melted and golden brown.

9. Remove from the oven and let it cool slightly. Garnish with fresh basil leaves.

10. Serve the Mediterranean Baked Eggplant with Tomato Sauce as a main dish or as a side dish with crusty bread or cooked rice.

Nutrition Facts:

- Serving Size: 1 serving
- Calories: 225
- Total Fat: 12g
- Saturated Fat: 3g
- Cholesterol: 9mg
- Sodium: 452mg
- Total Carbohydrate: 24g
- Dietary Fiber: 8g
- Sugars: 12g
- Protein: 9g

Please note that these nutrition facts are approximate and can vary based on the specific ingredients and brands used.

BROCCOLI AND QUINOA SALAD WITH LEMON-DIJON DRESSING

Preparation Time: 15 minutes Cooking Time: 15 minutes Serving: 4 servings

Ingredients:

- 1 cup quinoa
- 2 cups water
- 2 cups broccoli florets
- 1/2 red onion, thinly sliced

- 1/2 cup cherry tomatoes, halved
- 1/4 cup chopped fresh parsley
- 1/4 cup sliced almonds, toasted
- 1/4 cup dried cranberries
- Two tablespoons of lemon juice
- One tablespoon of Dijon mustard
- Two tablespoons extra-virgin olive oil
- Salt and pepper to taste

Directions:

1. Rinse the quinoa under cold water to remove any bitterness. In a saucepan, combine the quinoa and water. Bring to a boil, then reduce the heat and let it simmer for about 15 minutes. Remove from heat and let it cool.

2. In a large bowl, combine the cooked quinoa, broccoli florets, red onion, cherry tomatoes, chopped parsley, sliced almonds, and dried cranberries.

3. In a small bowl, whisk together the lemon juice, Dijon mustard, and extra-virgin olive oil. Season with salt and pepper.

4. Pour the dressing over the quinoa mixture and toss well to combine. Make sure all the ingredients are coated with the dressing.

5. Taste and adjust the seasoning if needed. You can add more lemon juice, mustard, salt, or pepper according to your preference.

6. Let the salad sit for about 10 minutes to allow the flavours to meld together. This will also give the broccoli a chance to soften slightly.

7. Serve the Broccoli and Quinoa Salad with Lemon-Dijon Dressing chilled or at room temperature. Garnish with additional sliced almonds and parsley if desired.

Nutrition Facts (per serving):

- Calories: 275
- Total Fat: 12g
- Saturated Fat: 1.5g
- Cholesterol: 0mg
- Sodium: 180mg
- Total Carbohydrate: 36g
- Dietary Fiber: 7g
- Sugars: 6g
- Protein: 9g

VEGAN LENTIL MEATLOAF

Preparation Time: 20 minutes Cooking Time: 1 hour Serving: 6 servings

Ingredients:

- 2 cups cooked green lentils
- One onion, finely chopped
- Two garlic cloves minced

- One carrot, grated
- One celery stalk, finely chopped
- One red bell pepper, finely chopped
- 1 cup breadcrumbs
- 1/2 cup ground flaxseed
- 1/4 cup nutritional yeast
- Two tablespoons of tomato paste
- Two tablespoons of soy sauce
- Two tablespoons of vegan Worcestershire sauce
- One tablespoon of Dijon mustard
- One tablespoon of dried oregano
- One tablespoon of dried thyme
- One tablespoon of smoked paprika
- Salt and pepper to taste

Directions:

1. Preheat the oven to 375°F (190°C) and line a loaf pan with parchment paper.
2. In a large bowl, mash the cooked lentils with a fork or potato masher until they're partially mashed but still have some texture.
3. Add the chopped onion, minced garlic, grated carrot, chopped celery, and chopped red bell pepper to the bowl. Mix well to combine.
4. Add the breadcrumbs, ground flaxseed, nutritional yeast, tomato paste, soy sauce, vegan Worcestershire sauce, Dijon mustard, dried oregano, dried thyme, smoked paprika, salt, and pepper to the bowl. Mix until all the ingredients are evenly distributed.

5. Transfer the lentil mixture to the prepared loaf pan and press it down firmly to pack it.

6. Bake in the preheated oven for 50-60 minutes or until the top is firm and golden brown.

7. Remove the lentil meatloaf from the oven and let it cool in the pan for about 10 minutes.

8. Carefully transfer the meatloaf to a cutting board and slice it into thick slices.

9. Serve the vegan lentil meatloaf slices with your favourite sides, such as mashed potatoes, roasted vegetables, or a side salad.

Nutrition Facts (per serving):

- Calories: 240
- Total Fat: 4.5g
- Saturated Fat: 0.6g
- Cholesterol: 0mg
- Sodium: 540mg
- Total Carbohydrate: 38g
- Dietary Fiber: 12g
- Sugars: 6g
- Protein: 13g

ZUCCHINI NOODLES WITH SPINACH PESTO

Preparation Time: 15 minutes Cooking Time: 10 minutes Servings: 4

Ingredients:

- Four medium zucchini
- 2 cups fresh spinach leaves
- 1/2 cup fresh basil leaves
- 1/4 cup pine nuts
- Three cloves garlic, minced
- 1/4 cup grated Parmesan cheese
- 1/4 cup extra-virgin olive oil
- Salt and pepper to taste
- Optional toppings: cherry tomatoes, grated Parmesan cheese, chopped fresh basil

Directions:

1. Wash the zucchini and trim off the ends. Using a spiralizer or a julienne peeler, create zucchini noodles. Set aside.

2. In a food processor, combine the spinach, basil, pine nuts, garlic, and Parmesan cheese. Pulse until the ingredients are well combined.

3. While the food processor is running, slowly drizzle in the olive oil until the mixture becomes smooth and creamy. Season with salt and pepper to taste.

4. Heat a large skillet over medium heat. Add the zucchini noodles and cook for about 3-4 minutes or until the noodles are slightly softened.

5. Remove the skillet from the heat and add the spinach pesto to the zucchini noodles. Toss well to coat the noodles evenly.

6. Divide the zucchini noodles with spinach pesto into serving bowls. Top with optional toppings like cherry tomatoes, grated Parmesan cheese, and chopped fresh basil.

7. Serve immediately and enjoy!

Nutrition Facts (per serving):

- Calories: 180
- Fat: 15g
- Carbohydrates: 8g
- Fibre: 3g
- Protein: 6g

SWEET POTATO AND BLACK BEAN QUESADILLAS

Preparation Time: 15 minutes Cooking Time: 25 minutes Servings: 4

Ingredients:

- Two medium sweet potatoes, peeled and diced
- One tablespoon of olive oil
- One small onion, diced
- Two cloves garlic, minced
- One teaspoon of ground cumin
- One teaspoon of chilli powder
- One can (15 ounces) of black beans, rinsed and drained

- Salt and pepper to taste
- Eight small flour tortillas
- 2 cups shredded cheese (cheddar or Monterey Jack)
- Optional toppings: salsa, sour cream, guacamole, chopped cilantro

Directions:

1. Place the diced sweet potatoes in a microwave-safe bowl. Cover with a damp paper towel and microwave on high for 5-6 minutes or until the sweet potatoes are tender. Set aside.

2. heat the olive oil over medium heat in a large skillet. Add the diced onion and minced garlic, and sauté until the onion becomes translucent, about 3-4 minutes.

3. Add the cooked sweet potatoes to the skillet, ground cumin, and chilli powder. Stir well to combine and cook for an additional 2-3 minutes.

4. Add the black beans to the skillet and season with salt and pepper to taste. Stir everything together and cook for another 2-3 minutes until heated through. Remove from heat and set aside.

5. Heat a separate skillet or griddle over medium heat. Place a tortilla on the skillet and sprinkle a layer of shredded cheese on half of the tortilla. Spoon a generous amount of the sweet potato and black bean mixture on top of the cheese.

6. Fold the tortilla in half to cover the filling and press down gently. Cook for 2-3 minutes on each side or until the tortilla is golden brown and the cheese has melted. Repeat with the remaining tortillas and filling.

7. Once cooked, transfer the quesadillas to a cutting board and let them cool for a minute. Cut each quesadilla into wedges.

8. Serve the Sweet Potato and Black Bean Quesadillas warm with your choice of toppings, such as salsa, sour cream, guacamole, or chopped cilantro.

Nutrition Facts (per serving): Calories: 320 Fat: 12g Carbohydrates: 43g Fiber: 9g Protein: 13g

Please note that the nutrition facts may vary depending on the specific ingredients and brands used.

CAULIFLOWER PIZZA CRUST WITH VEGGIE TOPPINGS

Preparation Time: 20 minutes Cooking Time: 30 minutes Serving: 4 servings

Ingredients: For the cauliflower crust:

- One medium-sized cauliflower head
- 1/2 cup grated Parmesan cheese
- 1/2 cup mozzarella cheese, shredded
- One teaspoon of dried oregano
- 1/2 teaspoon garlic powder
- Two eggs, lightly beaten
- Salt and pepper to taste

For the veggie toppings:

- 1/2 cup pizza sauce
- 1 cup shredded mozzarella cheese

- 1/2 cup sliced bell peppers
- 1/2 cup sliced mushrooms
- 1/4 cup sliced black olives
- 1/4 cup sliced red onions
- Fresh basil leaves for garnish

Directions:

1. Preheat your oven to 425°F (220°C).

2. Cut the cauliflower into florets and place them in a food processor. Pulse until the cauliflower resembles rice-like grains.

3. Transfer the cauliflower "rice" to a microwave-safe bowl and microwave on high for 4-5 minutes until cooked. Allow it to cool for a few minutes.

4. Place the cooked cauliflower in a clean kitchen towel and squeeze out as much moisture as possible. This step is crucial to get a crispy crust.

5. In a large mixing bowl, combine the cauliflower, grated Parmesan cheese, shredded mozzarella cheese, dried oregano, garlic powder, beaten eggs, salt, and pepper. Mix well until everything is evenly combined.

6. Line a baking sheet with parchment paper. Place the cauliflower mixture on the baking sheet and press it into a thin, round crust shape, about 1/4 inch thick.

7. Bake the cauliflower crust in the preheated oven for 15-20 minutes until it turns golden brown and crispy around the edges.

8. Remove the crust from the oven and let it cool for a few minutes. Leave the oven on.

9. Spread the pizza sauce evenly over the crust, leaving a small border around the edges. Sprinkle the shredded mozzarella cheese over the sauce.

10. Arrange the sliced bell peppers, mushrooms, black olives, and red onions over the cheese.

11. Place the pizza back in the oven and bake for an additional 10-12 minutes or until the cheese has melted and the toppings are cooked to your liking.

12. Remove the pizza from the oven and let it cool slightly. Garnish with fresh basil leaves.

13. Slice the cauliflower pizza into wedges and serve hot.

Nutrition Facts:

- Serving Size: 1 slice of pizza (based on four servings)
- Calories: Approximately 150 calories per slice
- Total Fat: 8g
- Saturated Fat: 4g
- Cholesterol: 85mg
- Sodium: 400mg
- Total Carbohydrate: 8g
- Dietary Fiber: 2g
- Sugars: 4g
- Protein: 12g

LENTIL AND VEGETABLE STIR-FRY WITH CASHEWS

Preparation Time: 15 minutes Cooking Time: 20 minutes Servings: 4

Ingredients:

- 1 cup lentils (green or brown), cooked
- Two tablespoons of vegetable oil
- One onion, thinly sliced
- 2 cloves garlic, minced
- 1 red bell pepper, thinly sliced
- One yellow bell pepper, thinly sliced
- 1 cup broccoli florets
- One carrot, thinly sliced
- 1 cup snow peas, ends trimmed
- 1/2 cup cashews
- Two tablespoons of soy sauce
- 1 tablespoon sesame oil
- 1 tablespoon rice vinegar
- One teaspoon of honey (optional)
- Salt and pepper to taste
- Sesame seeds for garnish (optional)

Directions:

1. Heat the vegetable oil in a large skillet or wok over medium heat.

2. Add the sliced onion and minced garlic to the skillet and sauté for 2-3 minutes until the onion becomes translucent.

3. Add the bell peppers, broccoli, carrot, and snow peas to the skillet. Stir-fry for 5-6 minutes until the vegetables are crisp-tender.

4. In the meantime, toast the cashews in a dry skillet over medium heat for 2-3 minutes until lightly golden. Set them aside.

5. Add the cooked lentils to the skillet and stir to combine with the vegetables.

6. In a small bowl, whisk together the soy sauce, sesame oil, rice vinegar, honey (if using), salt, and pepper.

7. Pour the sauce over the lentil and vegetable mixture and stir-fry for an additional 2-3 minutes until everything is coated and heated through.

8. Remove the skillet from heat and sprinkle the toasted cashews over the stir-fry.

9. Serve the Lentil and Vegetable Stir-Fry with Cashews hot, garnished with sesame seeds if desired.

Nutrition Facts (per serving):

- Calories: 320
- Total Fat: 16g
- Saturated Fat: 2.5g
- Cholesterol: 0mg
- Sodium: 650mg
- Total Carbohydrate: 33g
- Dietary Fiber: 8g
- Sugars: 7g
- Protein: 12g

- Vitamin D: 0%
- Calcium: 4%
- Iron: 15%
- Potassium: 10%

ROASTED BEET AND QUINOA SALAD WITH CITRUS DRESSING

Preparation Time: 20 minutes Cooking Time: 40 minutes Serving: 4

Ingredients:

- Two large beets peeled and cubed
- 1 cup quinoa
- 4 cups baby spinach
- One orange, peeled and segmented
- 1/4 cup chopped walnuts
- 1/4 cup crumbled feta cheese

For the Citrus Dressing:

- 1/4 cup fresh orange juice
- Two tablespoons of lemon juice
- One tablespoon honey
- Two tablespoons extra-virgin olive oil
- Salt and pepper to taste

Directions:

1. Preheat the oven to 400°F (200°C). Place the beet cubes on a baking sheet and drizzle with olive oil. Toss to coat evenly, then spread them out in a single layer. Roast for 30-40 minutes or until the beets are tender and slightly caramelized. Remove from the oven and let them cool.

2. In a medium saucepan, rinse the quinoa under cold water. Drain and add 2 cups of water to the saucepan. Bring to a boil over medium heat, then reduce the heat to low, cover, and simmer for 15-20 minutes or until the quinoa is cooked and the water is absorbed. Remove from heat and let it cool.

3. In a large salad bowl, combine the roasted beets, cooked quinoa, baby spinach, orange segments, chopped walnuts, and crumbled feta cheese.

4. In a small bowl, whisk together the orange juice, lemon juice, honey, olive oil, salt, and pepper to make the citrus dressing.

5. Pour the citrus dressing over the salad and toss gently to combine all the ingredients.

6. Serve the Roasted Beet and Quinoa Salad immediately and enjoy!

Nutrition Facts (per serving):

- Calories: 320
- Total Fat: 15g
- Saturated Fat: 3g
- Cholesterol: 8mg
- Sodium: 210mg
- Carbohydrates: 40g

- Fibre: 7g
- Sugar: 12g
- Protein: 9g

GRILLED PORTOBELLO MUSHROOM SANDWICH WITH ROASTED RED PEPPER AIOLI

Preparation Time: 15 minutes Cooking Time: 20 minutes Serving: 2 sandwiches

Ingredients:

- Two large Portobello mushrooms
- Four slices of bread (your choice of type)
- One red bell pepper
- 1/4 cup mayonnaise
- One clove of garlic, minced
- One tablespoon of lemon juice
- One tablespoon of olive oil
- Salt and pepper to taste
- Optional toppings: lettuce, tomato, avocado

Directions:

1. Preheat the grill or grill pan to medium-high heat.
2. Clean the Portobello mushrooms by wiping them with a damp cloth. Remove the stems and gently scrape out the gills using a spoon.

3. Place the mushrooms in a shallow dish and drizzle them with olive oil. Season with salt and pepper, ensuring both sides are coated.

4. Cut the red bell pepper in half, remove the seeds and stem, and brush the skin with olive oil.

5. Place the mushrooms and the red bell pepper halves on the grill. Cook for about 5 minutes on each side until the mushrooms are tender and the pepper skin is charred.

6. Remove the mushrooms and the red bell pepper from the grill. Let the mushrooms cool slightly, then slice them into thin strips.

7. Peel the charred skin off the red bell pepper and chop it into small pieces.

8. In a small bowl, combine the mayonnaise, minced garlic, lemon juice, and chopped red bell pepper. Mix well to create the roasted red pepper aioli.

9. Toast the slices of bread until golden and crisp.

10. Spread a generous amount of the roasted red pepper aioli on one side of each bread slice.

11. Layer the grilled Portobello mushroom slices on two slices of bread. Add optional toppings such as lettuce, tomato, and avocado if desired.

12. Top with the remaining two bread slices, aioli-side down, to create sandwiches.

13. Slice the sandwiches in half and serve immediately.

Nutrition Facts:

- The nutritional content may vary depending on the specific ingredients and quantities used.

Please note that the provided preparation time, cooking time, and servings are approximate and can be adjusted based on your preferences.

MEDITERRANEAN ROASTED VEGETABLES WITH HERBED QUINOA

Preparation Time: 15 minutes Cooking Time: 40 minutes Serving: 4

Ingredients: For the roasted vegetables:

- 1 medium eggplant, diced
- 2 zucchinis, sliced
- One red bell pepper, seeded and sliced
- One yellow bell pepper, seeded and sliced
- 1 red onion, thinly sliced
- 10 cherry tomatoes
- Three tablespoons olive oil
- Four cloves garlic, minced
- One teaspoon of dried oregano
- One teaspoon of dried basil
- Salt and pepper to taste

For the herbed quinoa:

- 1 cup quinoa
- 2 cups vegetable broth
- Two tablespoons fresh parsley chopped

- One tablespoon of fresh dill, chopped
- 1 tablespoon fresh mint, chopped
- Juice of 1 lemon
- Salt and pepper to taste

Directions:

1. Preheat your oven to 425°F (220°C).

2. In a large mixing bowl, combine the diced eggplant, sliced zucchini, red and yellow bell peppers, red onion, cherry tomatoes, olive oil, minced garlic, dried oregano, dried basil, salt, and pepper. Toss well to coat all the vegetables with the seasoning.

3. Spread the seasoned vegetables in a single layer on a baking sheet. Roast them in the preheated oven for about 30-35 minutes or until tender and slightly browned. Stir the vegetables once or twice during the cooking process for even roasting.

4. While the vegetables are roasting, prepare the herbed quinoa. Rinse the quinoa under cold water to remove any bitterness. In a medium saucepan, bring the vegetable broth to a boil. Add the rinsed quinoa, reduce the heat to low, cover the pan, and simmer for 15-20 minutes or until the quinoa is fluffy and the liquid is absorbed.

5. Once the quinoa is cooked, remove it from the heat and let it sit for 5 minutes. Fluff the quinoa with a fork and add the chopped parsley, dill, mint, lemon juice, salt, and pepper. Mix well to combine all the flavours.

6. When the roasted vegetables are ready, remove them from the oven and allow them to cool slightly.

7. To serve, divide the herbed quinoa among four plates or bowls. Top each serving with roasted Mediterranean vegetables.

Nutrition Facts (per serving):

- Calories: 270
- Total Fat: 10g
- Saturated Fat: 1g
- Cholesterol: 0mg
- Sodium: 450mg
- Carbohydrates: 40g
- Fibre: 9g
- Sugar: 10g
- Protein: 9g

CHICKPEA AND VEGETABLE STEW WITH TURMERIC

Preparation Time: 15 minutes Cooking Time: 30 minutes Serving: 4

Ingredients:

- Two tablespoons of olive oil
- 1 onion, chopped
- 3 cloves garlic, minced
- 1 teaspoon ground turmeric
- 1 teaspoon ground cumin
- 1 teaspoon paprika

- 1/2 teaspoon ground coriander
- 1/4 teaspoon cayenne pepper (optional for spiciness)
- Two carrots, peeled and diced
- Two bell peppers (any colour), diced
- 1 zucchini, diced
- 1 can (14 ounces) diced tomatoes
- One can (14 ounces) of chickpeas, drained and rinsed
- 2 cups vegetable broth
- Salt and pepper to taste
- Fresh cilantro, chopped (for garnish)

Directions:

1. Heat the olive oil in a large pot over medium heat. Add the chopped onion and minced garlic, and sauté until the onion becomes translucent about 5 minutes.

2. Stir in the ground turmeric, ground cumin, paprika, ground coriander, and cayenne pepper (if using). Cook for another minute to toast the spices and release their flavours.

3. Add the diced carrots, bell peppers, and zucchini to the pot. Cook for about 5 minutes, stirring occasionally, until the vegetables soften.

4. Pour in the diced tomatoes (with their juice), drained and rinsed chickpeas, and vegetable broth. Stir well to combine all the ingredients. Bring the stew to a boil, then reduce the heat to low.

5. Cover the pot and let the stew simmer for about 20 minutes or until the vegetables are tender. Season with salt and pepper to taste.

6. Once the stew is ready, spoon it into serving bowls. Garnish with freshly chopped cilantro.

Nutrition Facts (per serving):

- Calories: 240
- Fat: 8g
- Carbohydrates: 36g
- Fibre: 9g
- Protein: 9g

QUINOA AND AVOCADO SALAD WITH LIME-CILANTRO DRESSING

Preparation Time: 15 minutes Cooking Time: 15 minutes Serving: 4 servings

Ingredients:

- 1 cup quinoa
- 2 cups water
- One ripe avocado, diced
- 1 cup cherry tomatoes, halved
- 1/2 cup cucumber, diced
- 1/4 cup red onion, finely chopped
- 1/4 cup fresh cilantro, chopped
- Juice of 2 limes

- Two tablespoons of olive oil
- One clove of garlic, minced
- Salt and pepper to taste

Directions:

1. Rinse the quinoa under cold water using a fine-mesh sieve to remove bitterness. In a medium saucepan, combine the quinoa and water. Bring to a boil over medium-high heat.
2. Once boiling, reduce the heat to low, cover, and simmer for about 15 minutes or until the quinoa is tender and the water is absorbed. Remove from heat and let it cool.
3. In a large bowl, combine the cooked quinoa, diced avocado, cherry tomatoes, cucumber, red onion, and cilantro.
4. In a small bowl, whisk together the lime juice, olive oil, minced garlic, salt, and pepper to make the dressing.
5. Pour the lime-cilantro dressing over the quinoa mixture and toss gently to combine, ensuring all ingredients are well coated.
6. Taste and adjust the seasoning as needed. You can add more lime juice, salt, or pepper, according to your preference.
7. Let the salad sit for about 10 minutes to allow the flavours to meld together. Serve chilled.

Nutrition Facts (per serving):

- Calories: 280
- Fat: 14g
- Carbohydrates: 34g
- Fibre: 9g
- Protein: 7g

ZUCCHINI NOODLES WITH MUSHROOM BOLOGNESE SAUCE

Preparation Time: 15 minutes Cooking Time: 25 minutes Serving: 4 servings

Ingredients:

- 4 medium zucchini
- 2 tablespoons olive oil
- One onion, finely chopped
- Three cloves garlic, minced
- 8 ounces mushrooms, sliced
- 1 carrot, grated
- One red bell pepper, diced
- One can (14 ounces) of crushed tomatoes
- 2 tablespoons tomato paste
- One teaspoon of dried oregano
- One teaspoon of dried basil
- 1/2 teaspoon dried thyme
- Salt and pepper to taste
- Fresh basil leaves for garnish
- Grated Parmesan cheese for serving (optional)

Directions:

1. Using a spiralizer or a vegetable peeler, create zucchini noodles from the zucchini. Set aside.

2. Heat olive oil in a large skillet over medium heat. Add the chopped onion, minced garlic, and sauté until they become fragrant and translucent for about 2-3 minutes.

3. Add the sliced mushrooms, grated carrot, and diced bell pepper to the skillet. Cook for about 5 minutes or until the vegetables have softened.

4. Stir in the crushed tomatoes, tomato paste, dried oregano, dried basil, dried thyme, salt, and pepper. Reduce the heat to low and let the sauce simmer for 15 minutes, allowing the flavours to meld together.

5. While the sauce is simmering, heat another skillet over medium-high heat. Add the zucchini noodles and cook for about 2-3 minutes or until they are tender yet slightly crisp. Be careful not to overcook them.

6. Divide the zucchini noodles among four plates or bowls. Top each serving with a generous portion of the mushroom bolognese sauce.

7. Garnish with fresh basil leaves and sprinkle with grated Parmesan cheese, if desired.

Nutrition Facts (per serving): Calories: 180 Total Fat: 8g

- Saturated Fat: 1g
- Trans Fat: 0g Cholesterol: 0mg Sodium: 410mg Total Carbohydrate: 23g
- Dietary Fiber: 7g
- Sugars: 12g Protein: 6g

STUFFED SWEET POTATOES WITH LENTILS AND KALE

Preparation Time: 15 minutes Cooking Time: 1 hour Serving: 4 servings

Ingredients:

- 4 medium-sized sweet potatoes
- 1 cup cooked lentils
- 2 cups chopped kale
- One small onion, finely chopped
- Two cloves garlic, minced
- One tablespoon of olive oil
- One teaspoon of ground cumin
- 1/2 teaspoon paprika
- Salt and pepper to taste
- Optional toppings: chopped fresh parsley, grated Parmesan cheese

Directions:

1. Preheat the oven to 400°F (200°C).

2. Scrub the sweet potatoes thoroughly and pat them dry with a towel. Pierce each sweet potato several times with a fork.

3. Place the sweet potatoes on a baking sheet and bake for about 45-60 minutes or until they are tender when pierced with a fork.

4. While the sweet potatoes are baking, prepare the lentil and kale filling. Heat olive oil in a large skillet over medium heat.

5. Add the chopped onion and minced garlic to the skillet and sauté until the onion becomes translucent and the garlic is fragrant.

6. Stir in the ground cumin, paprika, salt, and pepper. Cook for another minute.

7. Add the chopped kale to the skillet and cook until it wilts and becomes tender, about 5-7 minutes.

8. Stir in the cooked lentils and cook for 2-3 minutes to heat through.

9. Once the sweet potatoes are done, remove them from the oven and let them cool slightly.

10. Slice each sweet potato lengthwise and gently fluff the flesh with a fork, creating a well for the filling.

11. Spoon the lentil and kale mixture into each sweet potato, distributing it evenly.

12. If desired, sprinkle with chopped fresh parsley and grated Parmesan cheese for added flavour.

13. Place the stuffed sweet potatoes back in the oven for another 5 minutes to warm up the filling.

14. Remove from the oven and serve hot.

Nutrition Facts (per serving):

- Calories: 320
- Fat: 5g
- Carbohydrates: 60g
- Fibre: 12g
- Protein: 12g

CAULIFLOWER BUFFALO WINGS WITH VEGAN RANCH DIP

Preparation Time: 15 minutes Cooking Time: 30 minutes Serving: 4

Ingredients: For Cauliflower Buffalo Wings:

- 1 head of cauliflower
- 1 cup all-purpose flour
- 1 cup unsweetened almond milk (or any plant-based milk)
- 1 teaspoon garlic powder
- One teaspoon paprika
- 1/2 teaspoon salt
- 1/4 teaspoon black pepper
- 1 cup buffalo hot sauce
- 2 tablespoons melted vegan butter

For Vegan Ranch Dip:

- 1 cup vegan mayonnaise
- 1/4 cup unsweetened almond milk (or any plant-based milk)
- 2 teaspoons apple cider vinegar
- 1 teaspoon dried dill
- One teaspoon of dried parsley
- 1/2 teaspoon garlic powder
- 1/2 teaspoon onion powder

- Salt and pepper to taste

Directions:

1. Preheat the oven to 450°F (230°C) and line a baking sheet with parchment paper.

2. Wash the cauliflower head and cut it into bite-sized florets, discarding the tough stem.

3. In a large bowl, whisk together the flour, almond milk, garlic powder, paprika, salt, and black pepper until smooth and well combined.

4. Dip each cauliflower floret into the batter, coating it evenly, and then place it on the prepared baking sheet. Repeat with all the florets.

5. Bake the cauliflower wings in the oven for 20 minutes or until they are crispy and golden brown.

6. While the cauliflower is baking, prepare the buffalo sauce by combining the buffalo hot sauce and melted vegan butter in a small bowl. Stir until well combined.

7. Once the cauliflower is cooked, remove it from the oven and let it cool for a few minutes. Then, dip each cauliflower wing into the buffalo sauce, coating it thoroughly. Place the coated wings back on the baking sheet.

8. Return the baking sheet to the oven and bake for 10 minutes or until the buffalo sauce is slightly caramelized.

9. While the cauliflower wings are baking for the second time, prepare the vegan ranch dip. In a small bowl, whisk together the vegan mayonnaise, almond milk, apple cider vinegar, dried dill, dried parsley, garlic powder, onion powder, salt, and pepper until well combined.

10. Once the cauliflower wings are done baking, remove them from the oven and let them cool for a few minutes. Serve them hot with the vegan ranch dip on the side.

Nutrition Facts: (Note: The following nutrition information is approximate and may vary depending on specific ingredients used)

Serving Size: 1/4 of the recipe Calories: 350 Total Fat: 20g Saturated Fat: 3g Trans Fat: 0g Cholesterol: 0mg Sodium: 1800mg Total Carbohydrate: 37g Dietary Fiber: 5g Total Sugars: 3g Protein: 6g

Enjoy your delicious Cauliflower Buffalo Wings with Vegan Ranch Dip!

LENTIL AND VEGETABLE CURRY WITH COCONUT MILK

Preparation Time: 15 minutes Cooking Time: 30 minutes Serving: 4 servings

Ingredients:

- 1 cup dried lentils
- Two tablespoons of vegetable oil
- One onion, chopped
- Three cloves garlic, minced
- 1 tablespoon grated ginger

- 1 tablespoon curry powder
- 1 teaspoon ground cumin
- One teaspoon of ground coriander
- 1/2 teaspoon turmeric powder
- 1/2 teaspoon chilli powder (optional, adjust to taste)
- 2 cups mixed vegetables (such as carrots, bell peppers, cauliflower, and peas), chopped
- One can (14 ounces) of coconut milk
- 1 cup vegetable broth
- Salt, to taste
- Fresh cilantro, chopped (for garnish)

Directions:

1. Rinse the lentils under cold water and drain.
2. Heat the vegetable oil in a large pot or Dutch oven over medium heat. Add the chopped onion and cook until softened about 5 minutes.
3. Add the minced garlic and grated ginger to the pot and cook for another minute until fragrant.
4. Stir in the curry powder, cumin, coriander, turmeric powder, and chilli powder (if using). Cook for about 1 minute to toast the spices and enhance their flavours.
5. Add the chopped vegetables to the pot and cook for 5 minutes, stirring occasionally.
6. Pour in the coconut milk and vegetable broth. Bring the mixture to a simmer.
7. Add the rinsed lentils to the pot and stir well to combine. Cover the pot and simmer for about 20 minutes or until the lentils and vegetables are tender.

8. Season with salt to taste. Adjust the seasoning and spices according to your preference.

9. Remove the pot from heat. Serve the lentil and vegetable curry over steamed rice or with naan bread.

10. Garnish with fresh chopped cilantro before serving.

Nutrition Facts (per serving):

- Calories: 320
- Fat: 17g
- Carbohydrates: 35g
- Fibre: 12g
- Protein: 11g

ROASTED BRUSSELS SPROUTS AND CHICKPEA SALAD WITH TAHINI DRESSING

Preparation Time: 15 minutes Cooking Time: 25 minutes Servings: 4

Ingredients:

- 1 pound Brussels sprouts, trimmed and halved
- 1 can chickpeas, drained and rinsed
- Two tablespoons of olive oil
- One teaspoon of ground cumin
- 1/2 teaspoon paprika

- Salt and black pepper, to taste
- 1/4 cup chopped fresh parsley
- 1/4 cup chopped fresh mint
- 1/4 cup chopped red onion

For the Tahini Dressing:

- 1/4 cup tahini
- Two tablespoons of lemon juice
- Two tablespoons water
- One garlic clove, minced
- 1/2 teaspoon ground cumin
- Salt and black pepper, to taste

Directions:

1. Preheat the oven to 425°F (220°C).

2. In a large bowl, combine the Brussels sprouts, chickpeas, olive oil, ground cumin, paprika, salt, and black pepper. Toss until the Brussels sprouts and chickpeas are evenly coated.

3. Spread the Brussels sprouts and chickpeas in a single layer on a baking sheet. Roast in the preheated oven for 20-25 minutes or until the Brussels sprouts are golden brown and crispy.

4. While the Brussels sprouts and chickpeas are roasting, prepare the tahini dressing. In a small bowl, whisk together the tahini, lemon juice, water, minced garlic, ground cumin, salt, and black pepper. Adjust the consistency by adding more water if needed.

5. Once the Brussels sprouts and chickpeas are done roasting, remove them from the oven and let them cool slightly.

6. In a large salad bowl, combine the roasted Brussels sprouts, chickpeas, chopped parsley, chopped mint, and chopped red

onion. Drizzle the tahini dressing over the salad and toss gently to combine.

7. Serve the roasted Brussels sprouts and chickpea salad immediately as a main dish or as a side dish with grilled chicken or fish.

Nutrition Facts (per serving):

- Calories: 260
- Total Fat: 15g
- Saturated Fat: 2g
- Cholesterol: 0mg
- Sodium: 190mg
- Total Carbohydrate: 25g
- Dietary Fiber: 8g
- Sugars: 4g
- Protein: 9g

VEGAN LENTIL BURGERS WITH SMOKY CHIPOTLE SAUCE

Preparation Time: 20 minutes Cooking Time: 30 minutes Serving: 4 burgers

Ingredients: For the lentil burgers:

- 1 cup cooked lentils
- 1/2 cup rolled oats
- 1/4 cup finely chopped onion
- Two cloves garlic, minced
- Two tablespoons ground flaxseed
- Three tablespoons water
- Two tablespoons of nutritional yeast
- One teaspoon of smoked paprika
- 1/2 teaspoon cumin
- Salt and pepper to taste
- 2 tablespoons olive oil (for cooking)

For the smoky chipotle sauce:

- 1/2 cup vegan mayonnaise
- One tablespoon of chipotle peppers in adobo sauce, minced
- One tablespoon of lime juice
- Salt to taste

Directions:

1. In a large mixing bowl, combine the cooked lentils, rolled oats, chopped onion, minced garlic, nutritional yeast, smoked paprika, cumin, salt, and pepper. Mix well.

2. In a small bowl, whisk together the ground flaxseed and water. Let it sit for a few minutes until it thickens and forms a gel-like consistency.

3. Add the flaxseed mixture to the lentil mixture and mix thoroughly until all the ingredients are evenly combined.

4. Shape the lentil mixture into four burger patties, pressing them firmly together. If the mixture feels too sticky, you can wet your hands with water to make it easier to handle.

5. Heat the olive oil in a skillet over medium heat. Place the lentil burgers in the skillet and cook for about 5-7 minutes on each side or until golden brown and crispy.

6. While the burgers are cooking, prepare the smoky chipotle sauce. In a small bowl, combine the vegan mayonnaise, minced chipotle peppers, lime juice, and salt. Mix well until all the ingredients are incorporated.

7. Once the lentil burgers are cooked, remove them from the skillet and let them cool slightly. Serve the burgers on buns or lettuce wraps, and top them with the smoky chipotle sauce.

Nutrition Facts (per serving):

- Calories: 320
- Fat: 16g
- Carbohydrates: 35g
- Protein: 12g
- Fibre: 8g
- Sodium: 480mg

Enjoy your Vegan Lentil Burgers with Smoky Chipotle Sauce!

QUINOA AND BLACK BEAN CHILI

Preparation Time: 15 minutes Cooking Time: 30 minutes Serving: 4

Ingredients:

- 1 cup quinoa, rinsed
- One tablespoon of olive oil
- One onion, diced
- Three cloves garlic, minced
- One red bell pepper, diced
- One green bell pepper, diced
- One can (14 ounces) of diced tomatoes
- One can (15 ounces) of black beans, drained and rinsed
- 1 can (15 ounces) of kidney beans, drained and rinsed
- 1 cup vegetable broth
- Two tablespoons chilli powder
- One tablespoon cumin
- 1 teaspoon smoked paprika
- Salt and pepper to taste
- Chopped fresh cilantro for garnish (optional)
- Lime wedges for serving (optional)

Directions:

1. In a medium-sized pot, bring 2 cups of water to a boil. Add the rinsed quinoa and cook according to package instructions. Once cooked, set aside.

2. Heat the olive oil over medium heat in a large pot or Dutch oven. Add the diced onion, minced garlic, and sauté until the onion is translucent and fragrant.

3. Add the diced red and green bell peppers to the pot and cook for another 3-4 minutes until they soften.

4. Pour in the diced tomatoes, black beans, kidney beans, and vegetable broth. Stir in the chilli powder, cumin, smoked paprika, salt, and pepper.

5. Bring the chilli to a boil, then reduce the heat to low. Cover the pot and let it simmer for about 20 minutes, allowing the flavours to meld together.

6. Once the chilli is cooked, add the cooked quinoa and stir to combine. Cook for an additional 5 minutes to heat the quinoa through.

7. Taste the chilli and adjust the seasoning if needed. If desired, garnish with chopped fresh cilantro.

8. Serve the quinoa and black bean chilli hot, with lime wedges on the side for squeezing over the chilli for added freshness and tang.

Nutrition Facts (per serving):

- Calories: 320
- Fat: 6g
- Carbohydrates: 55g
- Fibre: 15g
- Protein: 15g

ZUCCHINI NOODLES WITH CREAMY CASHEW SAUCE

Preparation Time: 15 minutes Cooking Time: 10 minutes Serving: 4 servings

Ingredients:

- Four medium-sized zucchini
- 1 cup raw cashews
- Two cloves garlic
- One tablespoon of nutritional yeast
- Two tablespoons of lemon juice
- 1/2 cup vegetable broth
- Salt and pepper to taste
- Fresh basil leaves for garnish (optional)

Directions:

1. Start by making creamy cashew sauce. Soak the cashews in water for at least 2 hours or overnight to soften them. Drain the cashews and rinse them well.

2. In a blender or food processor, combine the soaked cashews, garlic cloves, nutritional yeast, lemon juice, vegetable broth, salt, and pepper. Blend until smooth and creamy. If needed, add more vegetable broth to achieve the desired consistency. Set the sauce aside.

3. Using a spiralizer or a julienne peeler, make zucchini noodles out of the zucchini. Set aside.

4. Heat a large non-stick skillet over medium heat. Add the zucchini noodles and cook for about 3-4 minutes until they are slightly tender but retain some crunch.

5. Pour the creamy cashew sauce over the cooked zucchini noodles and toss gently to coat the noodles evenly. Continue cooking for another 1-2 minutes until the sauce is heated.

6. Remove the skillet from the heat and garnish with fresh basil leaves if desired.

7. Serve the zucchini noodles with creamy cashew sauce immediately as a main course or as a side dish.

Nutrition Facts (per serving):

- Calories: 280
- Total Fat: 18g
- Saturated Fat: 3g
- Sodium: 200mg
- Total Carbohydrate: 23g
- Dietary Fiber: 6g
- Sugars: 7g
- Protein: 10g

SWEET POTATO AND QUINOA STUFFED BELL PEPPERS

Preparation Time: 20 minutes Cooking Time: 40 minutes Servings: 4

Ingredients:

- 4 bell peppers (any colour)
- 1 cup quinoa, rinsed
- 2 cups vegetable broth
- Two medium sweet potatoes, peeled and diced
- One small onion, diced
- Two cloves garlic, minced
- One teaspoon of ground cumin
- One teaspoon paprika
- 1/2 teaspoon chilli powder
- Salt and pepper to taste
- 1/2 cup grated cheddar cheese (optional)
- Fresh parsley or cilantro, chopped (for garnish)

Directions:

1. Preheat the oven to 375°F (190°C). Slice off the tops of the bell peppers and remove the seeds and membranes. Set aside.

2. In a medium saucepan, combine the quinoa and vegetable broth. Bring to a boil, then reduce the heat to low, cover, and simmer for about 15 minutes or until the quinoa is cooked and the broth is absorbed. Remove from heat and set aside.

3. While the quinoa is cooking, heat some olive oil in a large skillet over medium heat. Add the diced sweet potatoes, onion, and minced garlic. Cook for about 5 minutes until the sweet potatoes are tender.

4. Stir in the ground cumin, paprika, chilli powder, salt, and pepper. Cook for an additional 2 minutes to allow the spices to blend.

5. Add the cooked quinoa to the skillet with the sweet potato mixture. Stir well to combine all the ingredients. Adjust the seasoning if needed.

6. Stuff each bell pepper with the sweet potato and quinoa mixture. Place the stuffed peppers in a baking dish. If desired, sprinkle grated cheddar cheese on top of each pepper.

7. Cover the baking dish with foil and bake in the preheated oven for 25-30 minutes or until the peppers are tender and the filling is heated through. If using cheese, remove the foil during the last 5 minutes of baking to allow it to melt and slightly brown.

8. Once cooked, remove the stuffed bell peppers from the oven and let them cool for a few minutes. Garnish with fresh parsley or cilantro before serving.

Nutrition Facts (per serving):

- Calories: 265
- Total Fat: 3.9g
- Saturated Fat: 1.7g
- Cholesterol: 7mg
- Sodium: 335mg
- Total Carbohydrate: 51.8g
- Dietary Fiber: 7.6g
- Sugars: 7.9g
- Protein: 7.6g

CAULIFLOWER AND CHICKPEA TACOS WITH LIME CREMA

Preparation Time: 15 minutes Cooking Time: 30 minutes Serving: 4

Ingredients: For the Cauliflower and Chickpea Filling:

- One small head of cauliflower, cut into small florets
- 1 can (15 ounces) chickpeas, rinsed and drained
- 2 tablespoons olive oil
- One teaspoon of ground cumin
- One teaspoon of chilli powder
- 1/2 teaspoon smoked paprika
- 1/2 teaspoon garlic powder
- Salt and pepper to taste

For the Lime Crema:

- 1/2 cup plain Greek yoghurt
- One tablespoon of lime juice
- One teaspoon of lime zest
- One tablespoon of chopped fresh cilantro
- Salt to taste

For Serving:

- 8 small corn tortillas
- 1 cup shredded lettuce
- 1/2 cup diced tomatoes
- 1/4 cup chopped red onion
- Fresh cilantro leaves for garnish

- Lime wedges for serving

Directions:

1. Preheat your oven to 425°F (220°C).

2. In a large bowl, combine the cauliflower florets, chickpeas, olive oil, cumin, chilli powder, smoked paprika, garlic powder, salt, and pepper. Toss until the cauliflower and chickpeas are evenly coated with the spices.

3. Spread the cauliflower and chickpea mixture on a baking sheet in a single layer. Roast in the preheated oven for about 25-30 minutes, or until the cauliflower is tender and golden brown, stirring once halfway through.

4. While the filling is roasting, prepare the lime crema. In a small bowl, combine the Greek yoghurt, lime juice, zest, chopped cilantro, and salt. Stir well to combine. Adjust the seasoning according to your taste.

5. Warm the corn tortillas in a dry skillet over medium heat until soft and pliable.

6. To assemble the tacos, spread a spoonful of the lime crema on each tortilla. Top with a generous amount of cauliflower and chickpea filling. Garnish with shredded lettuce, diced tomatoes, chopped red onion, and fresh cilantro leaves.

7. Serve the cauliflower and chickpea tacos with lime crema immediately with lime wedges on the side.

Nutrition Facts: (Per serving) Calories: 290 Fat: 9g Saturated Fat: 1.5g Cholesterol: 3mg Sodium: 250mg Carbohydrates: 43g Fiber: 9g Sugar: 5g Protein: 12g

LENTIL AND VEGETABLE SHEPHERD'S PIE

Preparation Time: 20 minutes Cooking Time: 45 minutes Serving: 6

Ingredients:

- 1 cup green lentils, rinsed
- 4 cups vegetable broth
- Two tablespoons of olive oil
- One large onion, chopped
- Three cloves garlic, minced
- Two carrots diced
- Two celery stalks, diced
- One red bell pepper, diced
- One zucchini, diced
- 1 cup frozen peas
- One tablespoon of tomato paste
- One teaspoon of dried thyme
- 1 teaspoon dried rosemary
- Salt and pepper to taste
- 4 cups mashed potatoes

Directions:

1. bring the vegetable broth to a boil in a large pot. Add the lentils and cook for 15-20 minutes or until tender. Drain any excess liquid and set aside.

2. Preheat your oven to 375°F (190°C).

3. heat the olive oil over medium heat in a separate large skillet. Add the onion and garlic and sauté until the onion becomes translucent and fragrant.

4. Add the carrots, celery, red bell pepper, zucchini, and peas to the skillet. Cook for about 5 minutes or until the vegetables are slightly tender.

5. Stir in the cooked lentils, tomato paste, dried thyme, rosemary, salt, and pepper. Cook for another 2 minutes, allowing the flavours to combine. Remove from heat.

6. Transfer the lentil and vegetable mixture to a baking dish and spread it out evenly.

7. Spread the mashed potatoes over the lentil and vegetable mixture, creating an even layer.

8. Place the baking dish in the preheated oven and bake for 20-25 minutes, or until the top is golden brown and the filling is bubbling.

9. Once cooked, remove from the oven and let it cool for a few minutes before serving.

Nutrition Facts (per serving):

- Calories: 350
- Fat: 8g
- Carbohydrates: 58g
- Fibre: 14g
- Protein: 14g

ROASTED VEGETABLE AND QUINOA STUFFED ZUCCHINI

Preparation Time: 20 minutes Cooking Time: 40 minutes Serving: 4 servings

Ingredients:

- Four medium zucchini
- 1 cup quinoa, rinsed
- 2 cups vegetable broth
- One red bell pepper, diced
- One yellow bell pepper, diced
- One small red onion, diced
- 2 cloves garlic, minced
- 1 cup cherry tomatoes, halved
- 1 tablespoon olive oil
- One teaspoon of dried oregano
- 1 teaspoon dried basil
- Salt and pepper to taste
- Fresh parsley for garnish

Directions:

1. Preheat the oven to 400°F (200°C). Cut the zucchini in half lengthwise and scoop out the flesh, leaving about 1/4 inch border. Reserve the flesh for later use.
2. In a medium saucepan, bring the vegetable broth to a boil. Add the quinoa and reduce the heat to low. Cover and simmer for 15-20 minutes or until the quinoa is cooked and

the broth is absorbed. Fluff the quinoa with a fork and set aside.

3. In a large skillet, heat the olive oil over medium heat. Add the red and yellow bell peppers, red onion, and minced garlic. Sauté for 5-7 minutes or until the vegetables are tender.
4. Meanwhile, chop the reserved zucchini flesh into small pieces. Add the chopped zucchini flesh and cherry tomatoes to the skillet. Season with dried oregano, dried basil, salt, and pepper. Cook for an additional 5 minutes, stirring occasionally.
5. In a large mixing bowl, combine the cooked quinoa and roasted vegetable mixture. Stir well to combine all the ingredients.
6. Place the hollowed zucchini halves on a baking sheet. Spoon the quinoa and vegetable mixture into each zucchini half, pressing it down gently.
7. Bake in the preheated oven for 20-25 minutes or until the zucchini is tender and the filling is heated through.
8. Remove from the oven and garnish with fresh parsley. Serve hot as a main dish or a side dish.

Nutrition Facts (per serving):

- Calories: 250
- Total Fat: 6g
- Saturated Fat: 1g
- Cholesterol: 0mg
- Sodium: 450mg
- Total Carbohydrate: 45g

- Dietary Fiber: 8g
- Sugars: 9g
- Protein: 9g

MEDITERRANEAN BAKED TOFU WITH COUSCOUS

Preparation Time: 15 minutes Cooking Time: 25 minutes Serving: 4

Ingredients:

- 1 block of firm tofu, drained and pressed
- One tablespoon of olive oil
- Two cloves garlic, minced
- One teaspoon of dried oregano
- One teaspoon of dried basil
- 1/2 teaspoon dried thyme
- 1/2 teaspoon paprika
- Salt and pepper to taste
- 1 cup couscous
- 1 1/2 cups vegetable broth
- 1 cup cherry tomatoes, halved
- 1/4 cup Kalamata olives, pitted and halved
- 1/4 cup crumbled feta cheese
- Fresh parsley, chopped (for garnish)

Directions:

1. Preheat your oven to 400°F (200°C). Line a baking sheet with parchment paper.
2. Slice the pressed tofu into 1/2-inch thick slices and place them on the prepared baking sheet.
3. In a small bowl, combine the olive oil, minced garlic, oregano, basil, thyme, paprika, salt, and pepper. Mix well.
4. Brush both sides of the tofu slices with the olive oil mixture, ensuring they are evenly coated.
5. Bake the tofu in the preheated oven for 20-25 minutes, flipping once halfway through, until the tofu is golden brown and crispy.
6. While the tofu is baking, prepare the couscous according to the package instructions, using vegetable broth instead of water for added flavour.
7. Once the couscous is cooked, fluff it with a fork and set aside.
8. In a large bowl, combine the cooked couscous, cherry tomatoes, Kalamata olives, and crumbled feta cheese. Toss gently to combine.
9. When the tofu is done, remove it from the oven and allow it to cool slightly. Cut the tofu slices into bite-sized pieces.
10. Add the tofu pieces to the couscous mixture and gently toss to combine all the ingredients.
11. Serve the Mediterranean baked tofu with couscous warm, garnished with fresh chopped parsley.

Nutrition Facts (per serving):

- Calories: 320
- Fat: 14g
- Carbohydrates: 29g

- Protein: 18g
- Fibre: 5g

BROCCOLI AND QUINOA STIR-FRY WITH TERIYAKI SAUCE

Preparation Time: 15 minutes Cooking Time: 20 minutes Serving: 4 servings

Ingredients:

- 1 cup quinoa
- 2 cups water
- Two tablespoons of vegetable oil
- Two cloves garlic, minced
- One small onion, diced
- 2 cups broccoli florets
- One red bell pepper, sliced
- One carrot, sliced
- 1 cup snap peas
- 1/4 cup low-sodium soy sauce
- 2 tablespoons teriyaki sauce
- One tablespoon of rice vinegar
- One tablespoon honey
- 1/2 teaspoon sesame oil
- 1/4 teaspoon red pepper flakes (optional)

- Sesame seeds, for garnish
- Chopped green onions for garnish

Directions:

1. Rinse the quinoa under cold water to remove any bitterness. In a saucepan, bring the water to a boil. Add the quinoa, reduce the heat to low, cover, and simmer for about 15 minutes or until the quinoa is tender and the water is absorbed. Remove from heat and let it sit for 5 minutes. Fluff with a fork.
2. Heat the vegetable oil over medium-high heat in a large skillet or wok. Add the minced garlic and diced onion. Sauté for 2-3 minutes until fragrant and the onion becomes translucent.
3. Add the broccoli florets, red bell pepper slices, carrot slices, and snap peas to the skillet. Stir-fry for about 5-6 minutes until the vegetables are tender-crisp.
4. In a small bowl, whisk together the soy sauce, teriyaki sauce, rice vinegar, honey, sesame oil, and red pepper flakes (if using). Pour the sauce over the stir-fried vegetables in the skillet. Stir well to coat the vegetables evenly. Cook for an additional 2-3 minutes until the sauce thickens slightly.
5. Add the cooked quinoa to the skillet and toss everything together until well combined. Cook for another 2-3 minutes to allow the flavours to meld together.
6. Remove from heat and garnish with sesame seeds and chopped green onions.
7. Serve the Broccoli and Quinoa Stir-Fry with Teriyaki Sauce hot as a main dish or a side dish.

Nutrition Facts: (Note: The following nutrition information is approximate and may vary depending on the specific ingredients used)

Serving Size: 1 serving Calories: 315 Total Fat: 10g Saturated Fat: 1.5g Cholesterol: 0mg Sodium: 650mg Total Carbohydrate: 49g Dietary Fiber: 7g Sugar: 10g Protein: 9g

Enjoy your Broccoli and Quinoa Stir-Fry with Teriyaki Sauce!

VEGAN LENTIL BOLOGNESE WITH SPAGHETTI SQUASH

Preparation Time: 15 minutes Cooking Time: 45 minutes Serving: 4

Ingredients:

- One medium spaghetti squash
- One tablespoon of olive oil
- One onion, finely chopped
- Two cloves garlic, minced
- One carrot, finely chopped
- One celery stalk, finely chopped
- One red bell pepper, finely chopped
- 1 cup dried lentils, rinsed and drained
- One can (14 ounces) of crushed tomatoes
- Two tablespoons of tomato paste
- One tablespoon of soy sauce
- One teaspoon of dried basil

- One teaspoon of dried oregano
- Salt and pepper to taste
- Fresh basil leaves, for garnish (optional)

Directions:

1. Preheat the oven to 400°F (200°C).
2. Cut the spaghetti squash in half lengthwise. Scoop out the seeds and pulp. Drizzle the cut sides with olive oil and sprinkle with salt and pepper. Place the squash halves, cut side down, on a baking sheet. Roast in the preheated oven for about 35-40 minutes or until the flesh is tender. Once cooked, use a fork to scrape the flesh into spaghetti-like strands. Set aside.
3. In a large saucepan, heat the olive oil over medium heat. Add the onion, garlic, carrot, celery, and red bell pepper. Sauté for 5-6 minutes or until the vegetables are tender.
4. Add the lentils, crushed tomatoes, tomato paste, soy sauce, dried basil, and dried oregano to the saucepan. Stir well to combine. Season with salt and pepper to taste.
5. Bring the mixture to a boil, then reduce the heat to low. Cover the saucepan and simmer for about 25-30 minutes or until the lentils are tender and the flavours have melded together.
6. To serve, divide the spaghetti squash strands among plates or bowls. Top with a generous scoop of the lentil bolognese sauce. Garnish with fresh basil leaves, if desired.
7. Enjoy your vegan lentil bolognese with spaghetti squash!

Nutrition Facts (per serving):

- Calories: 240
- Total Fat: 4g
- Saturated Fat: 0.5g
- Cholesterol: 0mg
- Sodium: 440mg
- Total Carbohydrate: 43g
- Dietary Fiber: 14g
- Sugars: 10g
- Protein: 12g
- Vitamin D: 0mcg
- Calcium: 100mg
- Iron: 4.5mg
- Potassium: 1030mg

ZUCCHINI NOODLES WITH PEANUT SAUCE AND TOFU

Preparation Time: 15 minutes Cooking Time: 15 minutes Serving: 4 servings

Ingredients:

- Four medium zucchini
- One block of firm tofu drained and cubed
- Two tablespoons of sesame oil
- Two cloves garlic, minced

- 1/4 cup creamy peanut butter
- Two tablespoons of soy sauce
- Two tablespoons of lime juice
- Two tablespoons of maple syrup
- 1/2 teaspoon red pepper flakes (optional)
- Two green onions, thinly sliced
- Two tablespoons chopped peanuts (optional)
- Fresh cilantro leaves for garnish

Directions:

1. Use a spiralizer or a vegetable peeler to turn the zucchini into noodles. Set aside.
2. Heat 1 tablespoon of sesame oil in a large skillet over medium-high heat. Add the tofu cubes and cook until golden brown on all sides. Remove from the skillet and set aside.
3. Add the remaining tablespoon of sesame oil and minced garlic in the same skillet. Sauté for 1-2 minutes until fragrant.
4. In a small bowl, whisk together peanut butter, soy sauce, lime juice, maple syrup, and red pepper flakes (if using). Add the sauce to the skillet and stir well to combine with the garlic.
5. Add the zucchini noodles to the skillet and toss to coat them in the peanut sauce. Cook for 2-3 minutes until the noodles are slightly softened.
6. Return the cooked tofu cubes to the skillet and gently toss them with the noodles and sauce.

7. Remove from heat and garnish with sliced green onions, chopped peanuts (if desired), and fresh cilantro leaves.
8. Serve immediately and enjoy!

Nutrition Facts (per serving):

- Calories: 275
- Fat: 17g
- Carbohydrates: 16g
- Fibre: 4g
- Protein: 15g
- Sugar: 9g
- Sodium: 390mg

STUFFED MUSHROOMS WITH LENTILS AND SUN-DRIED TOMATOES

Preparation Time: 15 minutes Cooking Time: 25 minutes Serving: 4

Ingredients:

- 12 large button mushrooms
- 1/2 cup cooked lentils
- 1/4 cup sun-dried tomatoes, chopped
- Two tablespoons of olive oil

- One small onion, finely chopped
- Two cloves garlic, minced
- 1/4 teaspoon dried thyme
- 1/4 teaspoon dried oregano
- Salt and pepper to taste
- 1/4 cup grated Parmesan cheese (optional)
- Fresh parsley, chopped (for garnish)

Directions:

1. Preheat the oven to 375°F (190°C). Line a baking sheet with parchment paper.
2. Remove the stems from the mushrooms and chop them finely. Set aside.
3. Heat the olive oil in a skillet over medium heat. Add the chopped onion and minced garlic. Sauté for 2-3 minutes until the onion becomes translucent.
4. Add the chopped mushroom stems, cooked lentils, and sun-dried tomatoes to the skillet. Stir in the dried thyme, dried oregano, salt, and pepper. Cook for an additional 3-4 minutes, allowing the flavours to combine.
5. Remove the skillet from heat and let the mixture cool slightly.
6. Spoon the lentil and sun-dried tomato mixture into the cavity of each mushroom, pressing it down gently. Place the stuffed mushrooms on the prepared baking sheet.
7. If desired, sprinkle grated Parmesan cheese over the stuffed mushrooms for an extra cheesy flavour.

8. Bake the mushrooms in the preheated oven for about 20-25 minutes or until the mushrooms are tender and the filling is golden brown.
9. Once cooked, remove the mushrooms from the oven and garnish with fresh chopped parsley.
10. Serve the stuffed mushrooms warm as an appetizer or a side dish. Enjoy!

Nutrition Facts (per serving):

- Calories: 120
- Total Fat: 6g
- Saturated Fat: 1g
- Cholesterol: 2mg
- Sodium: 150mg
- Total Carbohydrate: 12g
- Dietary Fiber: 4g
- Sugars: 3g
- Protein: 6g

CAULIFLOWER AND CHICKPEA COCONUT CURRY

Preparation Time: 15 minutes Cooking Time: 30 minutes Serving: 4 servings

Ingredients:

- One tablespoon of vegetable oil
- One medium onion, diced
- Three cloves garlic, minced
- One tablespoon of grated ginger
- One tablespoon of curry powder
- One teaspoon of ground cumin
- 1/2 teaspoon turmeric
- 1/2 teaspoon paprika
- 1/4 teaspoon cayenne pepper (optional for heat)
- One medium cauliflower, cut into florets
- One can (14 ounces) of chickpeas, drained and rinsed
- One can (14 ounces) of coconut milk
- 1 cup vegetable broth
- Two tablespoons of tomato paste
- One tablespoon of soy sauce
- One tablespoon of lime juice
- Salt and pepper, to taste
- Fresh cilantro, chopped (for garnish)
- Cooked rice or naan bread (for serving)

Directions:

1. Heat the vegetable oil in a large pot or Dutch oven over medium heat. Add the diced onion and sauté until translucent, about 5 minutes.
2. Add the minced garlic and grated ginger to the pot and cook for another 1-2 minutes, stirring occasionally.

3. In a small bowl, combine the curry powder, ground cumin, turmeric, paprika, and cayenne pepper (if using). Stir the spice mixture into the pot and cook for 1 minute to toast the spices.
4. Add the cauliflower florets and chickpeas to the pot, stirring to coat them with the spices. Cook for 2-3 minutes to slightly brown the cauliflower.
5. Pour in the coconut milk, vegetable broth, tomato paste, and soy sauce. Stir well to combine all the ingredients. Bring the mixture to a simmer and then reduce the heat to low. Cover the pot and let it cook for 20-25 minutes or until the cauliflower is tender.
6. Stir in the lime juice and season with salt and pepper to taste.
7. Serve the cauliflower and chickpea coconut curry over cooked rice or with naan bread. Garnish with fresh cilantro.

Nutrition Facts (per serving):

- Calories: 320
- Total Fat: 16g
- Saturated Fat: 11g
- Cholesterol: 0mg
- Sodium: 580mg
- Total Carbohydrate: 36g
- Dietary Fiber: 9g
- Sugars: 6g
- Protein: 10g

LENTIL AND VEGETABLE FRITTATA

Preparation Time: 15 minutes Cooking Time: 25 minutes Serving: 4 servings

Ingredients:

- 1 cup cooked lentils
- Six large eggs
- 1/4 cup milk
- One tablespoon of olive oil
- One small onion, diced
- One bell pepper, diced
- One zucchini, diced
- 1 cup sliced mushrooms
- Two cloves garlic, minced
- One teaspoon of dried thyme
- Salt and pepper to taste
- 1/2 cup shredded cheddar cheese

Directions:

1. Preheat your oven to 375°F (190°C).
2. Whisk together the eggs, milk, salt, and pepper in a large bowl. Set aside.
3. Heat olive oil in a large oven-safe skillet over medium heat. Add the onion, bell pepper, zucchini, mushrooms, garlic, dried thyme, salt, and pepper. Sauté for about 5 minutes until the vegetables are tender.

4. Add the cooked lentils to the skillet and stir to combine them with the vegetables.
5. Pour the egg mixture over the vegetables and lentils in the skillet. Stir gently to distribute the ingredients evenly.
6. Sprinkle the shredded cheddar cheese on top of the frittata.
7. Transfer the skillet to the preheated oven and bake for 20-25 minutes until the eggs are set and the cheese is melted and golden brown.
8. Once cooked, remove the skillet from the oven and let the frittata cool for a few minutes.
9. Slice the frittata into wedges and serve warm.

Nutrition Facts (per serving):

- Calories: 250
- Total Fat: 12g
- Saturated Fat: 4.5g
- Cholesterol: 250mg
- Sodium: 350mg
- Carbohydrates: 19g
- Fibre: 5g
- Sugars: 4g
- Protein: 18g

GRILLED PORTOBELLO MUSHROOM SALAD WITH BALSAMIC GLAZE

Preparation Time: 15 minutes Cooking Time: 15 minutes Serving: 4 servings

Ingredients:

- Four large Portobello mushrooms
- Two tablespoons of olive oil
- Salt and pepper, to taste
- 4 cups mixed salad greens
- 1 cup cherry tomatoes, halved
- 1/2 cup red onion, thinly sliced
- 1/4 cup crumbled feta cheese
- Two tablespoons fresh basil chopped
- Balsamic glaze for drizzling

Directions:

1. Preheat the grill to medium-high heat.
2. Clean the Portobello mushrooms by removing the stems and gently brushing off any dirt. Do not wash them, as they can absorb water.
3. In a small bowl, whisk together the olive oil, salt, and pepper. Brush the mixture evenly over both sides of the mushrooms.
4. Place the mushrooms on the preheated grill, gill side down. Grill for about 5-7 minutes per side or until the mushrooms are tender and grill marks appear.

5. Once grilled, remove the mushrooms from the grill and let them cool slightly. Slice them into thin strips.
6. In a large salad bowl, combine the mixed salad greens, cherry tomatoes, red onion, feta cheese, and fresh basil.
7. Add the sliced grilled Portobello mushrooms to the salad bowl.
8. Drizzle the salad with balsamic glaze.
9. Toss the salad gently until all the ingredients are well combined.
10. Serve the Grilled Portobello Mushroom Salad immediately, and enjoy!

Nutrition Facts: (Note: Nutritional values may vary depending on the specific ingredients used and serving size)

- Serving Size: 1 serving
- Calories: 180
- Total Fat: 12g
- Saturated Fat: 3g
- Cholesterol: 8mg
- Sodium: 290mg
- Total Carbohydrate: 15g
- Dietary Fiber: 4g
- Sugars: 7g
- Protein: 6g

Please note that the nutrition facts are approximate and can vary based on the ingredients used.

QUINOA AND BLACK BEAN STUFFED ZUCCHINI BOATS

Preparation Time: 20 minutes Cooking Time: 30 minutes Serving: 4 servings

Ingredients:

- Four medium-sized zucchini
- 1 cup cooked quinoa
- 1 cup black beans, rinsed and drained
- One small onion, diced
- Two cloves garlic, minced
- One red bell pepper, diced
- 1/2 cup corn kernels (fresh or frozen)
- One teaspoon cumin
- One teaspoon of chilli powder
- 1/2 teaspoon paprika
- Salt and pepper to taste
- 1 cup shredded cheese (cheddar or Mexican blend)
- Fresh cilantro, chopped (for garnish)

Directions:

1. Preheat the oven to 375°F (190°C).

2. Cut the zucchini in half lengthwise. Use a spoon to scoop out the flesh, leaving a 1/4-inch thick shell. Chop the scooped-out zucchini flesh and set it aside.
3. In a large skillet, heat some oil over medium heat. Add the onion, garlic, and sauté until they become translucent and fragrant.
4. Add the chopped zucchini flesh, red bell pepper, and corn kernels to the skillet. Cook for about 5 minutes until the vegetables are tender.
5. Stir in the cooked quinoa, black beans, cumin, chilli powder, paprika, salt, and pepper. Cook for an additional 2-3 minutes to allow the flavours to blend.
6. Place the zucchini boats in a baking dish. Spoon the quinoa and black bean mixture into each boat, dividing it evenly.
7. Cover the baking dish with foil and bake for 20 minutes.
8. Remove the foil, sprinkle the shredded cheese over the stuffed zucchini boats, and return to the oven. Bake for an additional 10 minutes or until the cheese is melted and bubbly.
9. Remove from the oven and let it cool slightly. Garnish with fresh chopped cilantro.
10. Serve the quinoa and black bean stuffed zucchini boats as a main or side dish. Enjoy!

Nutrition Facts: (Note: The following nutrition facts are approximate and may vary based on the specific ingredients used.)

Serving Size: 1 stuffed zucchini boat Calories: 220 Total Fat: 7g Saturated Fat: 3.5g Cholesterol: 20mg Sodium: 350mg Total Carbohydrate: 30g Dietary Fiber: 7g Total Sugars: 5g Protein: 11g

Please note that these nutrition facts are estimated and can vary depending on the specific brands and quantities of ingredients used.

ZUCCHINI NOODLES WITH LEMON GARLIC SHRIMP

Preparation Time: 15 minutes Cooking Time: 10 minutes Serving: 2 servings

Ingredients:

- Two medium-sized zucchini
- 8-10 large shrimp, peeled and deveined
- Two tablespoons of olive oil
- Three cloves garlic, minced
- One teaspoon of lemon zest
- Two tablespoons of lemon juice
- Salt and pepper to taste
- Fresh parsley, chopped (for garnish)

Directions:

1. Using a spiralizer or a julienne peeler, create zucchini noodles from the zucchini. Set aside.

2. Heat one tablespoon of olive oil over medium-high heat in a large skillet.
3. Add the shrimp to the skillet and cook for 2-3 minutes on each side until they turn pink. Remove the shrimp from the skillet and set aside.
4. Add the remaining tablespoon of olive oil and minced garlic in the same skillet. Sauté for about 1 minute until fragrant.
5. Add the zucchini noodles to the skillet and sauté for 2-3 minutes until they are tender but still have a slight crunch. Be careful not to overcook them.
6. Return the cooked shrimp to the skillet with the zucchini noodles.
7. Add lemon zest, lemon juice, salt, and pepper to the skillet. Toss everything together to combine well and cook for an additional minute to heat through.
8. Remove from heat and garnish with fresh parsley.
9. Serve the zucchini noodles with lemon garlic shrimp immediately while they are still warm.

Nutrition Facts (per serving):

- Calories: 210
- Fat: 11g
- Carbohydrates: 10g
- Protein: 18g
- Fibre: 3g

CONCLUSION

Congratulations on completing the "Pegan Diet Cookbook for Beginners: 1000-Days of Mouthwatering, Delicious Recipes, Meal Plans, and Practical Tips for Beginners to Achieve Optimal Health and Sustainable Weight Loss." We hope this cookbook has provided you with a wealth of knowledge, inspiration, and practical guidance on your Pegan journey.

Throughout this cookbook, we have explored the concept of the Pegan diet, which combines the best elements of the Paleo and vegan diets to create a balanced and nutritious eating plan. By following the Pegan diet, you have taken a proactive step towards improving your health, nourishing your body, and achieving sustainable weight loss.

We have included a wide variety of recipes that cater to different tastes and dietary preferences. From vibrant salads and hearty soups to flavorful main courses and indulgent desserts, these recipes have been carefully crafted to ensure a harmonious blend of flavours, textures, and nutrients. We hope you have enjoyed preparing and savouring these mouthwatering dishes as much as we have enjoyed creating them.

In addition to the delicious recipes, we have provided practical tips and guidance to support your Pegan journey. From meal planning and grocery shopping to food substitutions and maintaining a balanced lifestyle, these tips will help you navigate the challenges that may arise while adopting a new eating plan.

Remember, it's all about finding a sustainable approach that works for you and fits seamlessly into your daily routine.

As you continue your Pegan journey, we encourage you to embrace the principles of the Pegan diet beyond the recipes in this cookbook. Focus on consuming whole, unprocessed foods, emphasizing fruits, vegetables, lean proteins, healthy fats, and high-quality carbohydrates. Strive to choose organic, locally sourced ingredients whenever possible, and listen to your body's hunger and satiety cues.

Remember that optimal health is a lifelong journey, and the Pegan diet is just one piece of the puzzle. Engage in regular physical activity, prioritize sleep and stress management, and nurture your mental and emotional well-being. By adopting a holistic approach to health, you'll maximize the benefits of the Pegan diet and create a sustainable and fulfilling lifestyle.

We hope this cookbook has empowered you to take charge of your health, experiment with new flavours, and enjoy the pleasures of cooking and eating delicious Pegan meals. Your culinary journey doesn't end here – continue to explore, innovate, and adapt the Pegan diet principles to suit your tastes and needs.

Thank you for choosing the "Pegan Diet Cookbook for Beginners," and we wish you an abundance of health, happiness, and culinary adventures on your Pegan journey.

Bon appétit and happy Pegan cooking!

Made in the USA
Columbia, SC
18 October 2024